COCHLEAR IMPLANTS

What Parents Should Know

COCHLEAR IMPLANTS
What Parents Should Know

Betty Loy and Peter Roland

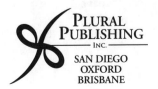

PLURAL
PUBLISHING
INC.

SAN DIEGO
OXFORD
BRISBANE

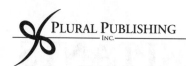

PLURAL PUBLISHING
INC.

5521 Ruffin Road
San Diego, CA 92123

e-mail: info@pluralpublishing.com
Web site: http://www.pluralpublishing.com

49 Bath Street
Abingdon, Oxfordshire OX14 1EA
United Kingdom

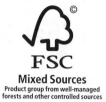

FSC
Mixed Sources
Product group from well-managed
forests and other controlled sources

Cert no. SW-COC-002283
www.fsc.org
© 1996 Forest Stewardship Council

Typeset in 11/12 Garamond by Flanagan's Publishing Services, Inc.
Printed in the United States of America by McNaughton and Gunn, Inc.

Library of Congress Cataloging-in-Publication Data:

Loy, Betty.
  Cochlear implants : what parents should know / Betty Loy and Peter Roland.
      p. cm.
  Includes index.
  ISBN-13: 978-1-59756-296-6 (alk. paper)
  ISBN-10: 1-59756-296-3 (alk. paper)
  1. Cochlear implants—Popular works. I. Roland, Peter S. II. Title.
  RF305.L693 2008
  617.8'8220592—dc22
                                                                  2008030143

Contents

Acknowledgments

This book was prepared entirely while the authors were affiliated with the Dallas Cochlear Implant Program and the institutions supporting it: the University of Texas Southwestern Medical Center, the University of Texas at Dallas Callier Center for Communication Disorders and the Advanced Hearing Research Center, and Children's Medical Center of Dallas.

We would like to thank Janette Cantwell, mother of Megan, and Amy Fields, mother of Andrew, and other mothers and fathers who graciously took the time to read chapters in the book and offer their sterling advice for improvement. We are also grateful to the many families who let us use pictures of their children in various aspects of the cochlear implant process.

All of the children pictured in the book have at least one cochlear implant. We would like to thank their parents for allowing them to participate and to thank them by name: Megan Cantwell, Jordan Capener, Andrew Cobb, Emma Cook, Charles Cooper, Andrew Fields, Trenton Holland, Jared Hughes, Logan Hupp, John McPherson, Todd McPherson, Ben Purcel, Katherine Ramirez, Sir Wesley (Scooter) Raven, and Emily Tranchina.

Our gratitude is heartily extended to Melissa Sweeney, certified auditory-verbal therapist, speech-language pathologist, author of this book's Chapter 8, and an essential partner in the creation and completion of the entire project.

We would like to express our thanks to Ashley House, Jill Rule, and Paige Duke for their incomparable assistance with document gathering, formatting, and organizational skills. Their collective sense of humor was of great help too.

The writing of Chapter 7 was partially supported by Grant Number KL2RR024983, titled, "North and Central Texas Clinical and Translational Science Initiative" (Milton Packer, MD, PI) from the National Center for Research Resources (NCRR), a component of the National Institutes of Health (NIH), and NIH Roadmap for Medical Research, and its contents are solely the responsibility of the author and do not necessarily represent the official views of the NCRR or NIH. Information on NCRR is available at http://www.ncrr.nih.gov/

We are grateful to Emily Perl Kingsley for granting permission to reprint "Welcome to Holland" in Chapter 9. This simple essay brings clarity and perspective to parents of special needs children around the world and has since she wrote it in 1987.

The writing of Chapter 10 was supported, in part, by Grant Numbers RO1-DC03100 and RO1-DC008335 from the National Institute on Deafness and Other Communication Disorders (NIDCD) of the National Institutes of Health. We gratefully acknowledge the families of children with implants from across the United States and Canada who enthusiastically participated in this study. Our appreciation is extended to Jean Moog and Karen Stein of the Moog Center for Deaf Education for thoughtful editing of this manuscript.

Our program has components in three distinct institutions. While all are on the same campus, the navigation from one service provider to another, say, from the surgeon's office to the speech pathologist's office, can prove to be a daunting task. We'd like to thank all those people who help our families get from one office to another, from one end of the process to the other, and in all other ways offer encouragement and support. There could be no program and, therefore, no guide book without them.

Introduction

This handbook was written by members of the Dallas Cochlear Implant Program (DCIP). The program is a collaborative venture of the University of Texas Southwestern Medical Center, the University of Texas at Dallas Callier Center for Communication Disorders and the Advanced Hearing Research Center, and Children's Medical Center of Dallas. The DCIP delivers medical, surgical, therapeutic, and counseling services to families seeking cochlear implantation and has done so since 1986.

This is a book about the world of cochlear implants, hearing, and speaking. The idea for this handbook came to us from parents we've been fortunate to meet and work with in our program.

Parents need information they can rely on to make informed decisions, and they need it in a convenient, easy to understand format. Although information is everywhere, it is nearly impossible to assemble the necessary knowledge in one place in order to make wise choices. Our task, therefore, was to gather pertinent information about deafness and cochlear implantation from recognized experts and organize it in a useable way.

With this book as a guide, you begin your journey into the world of deafness, a place you didn't know you were going. If you are a hearing person from a traditionally hearing family you are about to expand your vocabulary, learn anatomy and physiology of the head and, particularly, the ear, and meet specialists you didn't know existed like audiologists and speech pathologists and special educators and early childhood learning specialists and so on. By the time you are through (although you never really are through) you will have what seems like a college degree majoring in hearing loss, hearing habilitation, grief survival, speech and language development, and childhood education advocacy and a minor in electronics, battery life, and magnet strength. If you are deaf or are otherwise a member of the Deaf community, you are already wise to many of the things your hearing comrades are about to learn. In the world of cochlear implantation, though, there are additional things everyone needs to add to his or her hearing knowledge. In the rapidly changing world of medical technology, no one book can have all the information for all time, but what has been written here offers a solid foundation regardless of your starting point.

When seeking advice, wisdom leads us to those who have much experience with the question at hand. Helen Keller, arguably the best known and most admired deaf (and blind) person in American culture, wrote to a friend, " . . . after a lifetime in silence and darkness to be deaf is a greater affliction than to be blind. . . . Hearing is the soul of knowledge and information on a high order. To be cut off from hearing is to be isolated indeed" (Love, 1933).

It may seem obvious to you that hearing and speaking are preferable to the alternative, but it is not the choice all make when faced with this decision. The DCIP approaches cochlear implantation with the bias that it is better to hear than not, that hearing is necessary for normal language and speech development, and that parents alone have the right to make this decision on behalf of their child.

Betty Loy
Peter Roland
Dallas, Texas

Reference

Love, J. K. (1933). *Helen Keller in Scotland: A personal record written by herself.* London: Methuen & Company.

Contributors

Lindsay Bondurant, MS, CCC-A
University of Texas at Dallas
Callier Center for Communication
   Disorders
Dallas, Texas
Chapter 9

Ann E. Geers, PhD
Adjunct Professor
University of Texas at Dallas
Callier Center for Communication
   Disorders
Dallas, Texas
Chapter 10

Christine H. Gustus, MS, CCC-SLP
Director of Admissions and
   Evaluations
Missouri Center for Deaf Education
St. Louis, Missouri
Chapter 10

Betty Loy, AuD, CCC-A, FAAA
Clinical Research Manager
Department of Otolaryngology-Head
   and Neck Surgery
Special Assistant to the Board of
   Directors
Dallas Cochlear Implant Program
University of Texas Southwestern
   Medical Center
Dallas, Texas
Chapter 1

Marjorie K. Maier, MSW, MBA
Department of Otolaryngology-Head
   and Neck Surgery

University of Texas Southwestern
   Medical Center
Dallas, Texas
Chapter 4

Peter S. Roland, MD
Professor and Chairman
Department of
   Otolaryngology/Head and Neck
   Surgery
University of Texas Southwestern
   Medical Center
Dallas, Texas
Holder of the Arthur E. Meyerhoff
   Chair in Otolaryngology/Head
   and Neck Surgery
Chapter 6

Jessica Sullivan
Advanced Hearing Research Center
University of Texas at Dallas
Callier Center for Communication
   Disorders
Dallas, Texas
Chapter 9

**Melissa H. Sweeney, MS, CCC-SLP,
   LSLS Cert. AVT**
Cochlear Implant Program Manager
Speech-Language Pathologist
Certified Auditory-Verbal Therapist
University of Texas at Dallas
Callier Center for Communication
   Disorders
Dallas, Texas
Chapter 8

Linda Thibodeau, PhD
Professor and Head, AuD Program
Advanced Hearing Research Center
University of Texas at Dallas
Callier Center for Communication
    Disorders
Dallas, Texas
Chapter 9

Emily Tobey, PhD
Professor and Nelle C. Johnston
    Chair
Advanced Hearing Research Center
University of Texas at Dallas
Callier Center for Communication
    Disorders
Dallas, Texas
Chapter 2

**Pamela Tunney-Kruger, AuD,
    CCC-A**
Audiologist/Faculty Associate
University of Texas Southwestern
    Medical Center
Dallas, Texas
Chapter 3

**Andrea D. Warner-Czyz, PhD,
    CCC-A**
Research Associate
Advanced Hearing Research Center
University of Texas at Dallas
Callier Center for Communication
    Disorders
Dallas, Texas
Chapter 7

Holly S. Whalen, AuD, CCC-A
Audiologist
University of Texas at Dallas
Callier Center for Communication
    Disorders
Dallas, Texas
Chapter 5

Phillip L. Wilson, AuD, CCC-A
Head of Audiology
University of Texas at Dallas
Callier Center for Communication
    Disorders
Dallas, Texas
Chapter 5

This book is dedicated to parents and caregivers of deaf children everywhere. Nothing is more precious than our children, and few things are more difficult than raising a special needs child. By this dedication we gratefully acknowledge your sacrifices, your strength and courage, and above all your willingness to share your stories in order to help others.

Chapter 1

Upon Learning Your Child Can't Hear

By Betty Loy

You are not alone. Every day, 33 babies are born with a hearing loss in this country, eight or nine of them with a loss so profound they hear nothing at all. Every day, when parents are given this news, they join the thousands of other families whose lives are changed forever.

There may be a sense of loneliness, though, as it dawns on you what lies ahead. Not only is your emotional life in turmoil and needing attention, you must become an expert in deafness, hearing aids, cochlear implants, and speech and language development. You and your family will continue to be under a great deal of stress and that puts you at risk for additional family problems. Do you have the strength? Do you have the resources, including money? As you begin dealing with feelings you never thought you would have and making decisions you never dreamed you'd have to make, you may feel very alone. We will talk about strategies for coping with this feeling later in the chapter.

For now, please take comfort in the undisputable fact that others, no stronger than you, no smarter than you, and no less heartbroken than you, have successfully made it to the other side of this news with self and family intact. In your community, there are families who have chosen the cochlear implant (CI) for their child; they have experienced the many ups and downs of the process and are well into what I call their CI life. Find them! Listening to their stories and having them listen to yours will help you bring shape and form to your feelings and give you back some of your power. Even if you choose an option other than an implant, they can be helpful, a source of friendship, inspiration, and advice. If no other family lives close enough to offer assistance, please refer to the list of resources in the back of this book to find a CI community of support, either on-line, by phone, or by mail.

In addition to the many families who share your acquaintance with deafness, there are others who are prepared to help you when you are ready—the cochlear implantation specialists. A typical CI team consists of these professionals:

- Otolaryngology (ENT) physicians
- Audiologists
- Speech-language pathologists with auditory-verbal certification
- Language interpreters
- Insurance experts
- Social workers/case managers

Our doctors have many names. Physicians known as ear, nose, and throat (ENT) doctors, otologists, otolaryngologists, and neurotologists all specialize in diseases of the ear, nose, and throat. Most ENT specialists don't perform CI surgery, though, and are not experts in cochlear implantation. When you discuss your child's condition with a physician, be sure he or she is an expert in CI and has surgical experience.

The next specialist is probably less familiar to you: an audiologist. The audiologist specializes in performing diagnostic hearing tests and working with you and your child after implantation. The specialist who works with evaluating your child's speech and language development and providing treatment is the speech-language pathologist. Depending on your child's age and needs, you may or may not work with the speech pathologist after implantation, but your child will be evaluated prior to the CI surgery in order for the team to have baseline information about your child's level of language development.

If your child is old enough, there might be a need for an evaluation by a psychologist. The CI team needs to know if there are any conditions that might interfere with the success of an implant.

If your child or any family member uses sign language, there should be an interpreter on the team so that all present during team/family meetings can participate.

Finally, there should be one team member's name and number you can contact at any time during the CI process to answer questions and direct your concerns to the appropriate team member. This person is usually called the case manager and often is trained as a social worker. All of these people chose hearing and speech disorders to be their life's work. They are dedicated to working with families during this daunting experience to make it easier and less lonely through their learning, service, and caring. Because of them, you don't have to make decisions uninformed or walk through the maze of doctor visits, testing, and surgery alone. Every step of the way, you should have someone to reach out to for information, help, and advice. The message is clear: you don't have to be alone and you shouldn't be. In fact, if your CI team doesn't put you in the center and make you feel important and gain your complete confidence, get another team.

Grief

Grief is a normal response to loss. While there is no way to predict how your grief will show itself, I know you are experiencing it. As you know by now, grief is not a single emotion but a combination of anger, guilt, yearning, fear, depression, and other feelings that rise and fall and rise again. Grieving has been referred to as a cycle, but hardly a perfect one (Clark & English, 2004). Dealing with your grief is like climbing a mountain, and a slippery one at that. You may find yourself close to the top one day, close to overcoming your despair; and the next you're halfway down again, tumbling back to feelings you thought you'd successfully beaten. The other members of your family are scrambling all over this mountain too, trying to gain their own footing and balance. No two people grieve in exactly the same way because what has been lost is not the same for everyone. You may be feeling denial, while your hearing child is feeling angry at being left out of the conversation or sad about your being sad. This may be the first serious crisis you've had to face, the first critical juncture with your spouse or partner.

Parents have reported to us "gripping and paralyzing" emotional roller coaster rides, controlling them totally at first. Over time, the wild emotional swings lessen as they regain confidence through knowledge, counseling, love of family and friends, their faith, and the support of the professionals around them. As certain milestones (set by you) are met, stress is reduced step by step. Grieving is a process, and it takes work and time.

The culmination of grief is acceptance. Eventually, you will get to a point of accepting the deafness of your child as just another part of who he is. This doesn't mean everything is okay, no more worries, or that things are back to normal. Rather, arriving at this stage of acceptance means you are no longer depressed, or angry, or bargaining for a different result (Kubler-Ross, 1969). Acceptance means that yearning for what you thought you had lost is over, replaced by the joy of knowing what you have. Acceptance is not erasing the loss, but transcending it (Bristor, 1984), rising above the devastation to a new level of living.

Not all couples of special needs children experience a high level of grief and anger; it is not automatic. One mother stated she felt almost as though something was wrong with her reaction to her son's deafness because other parents seemed to be grieving so much more than she and her husband. She attributes this sense of early acceptance to her faith and her realization that her son was exactly who and where he was supposed to be.

If you are not yet at the acceptance stage, you might be asking how to cope with this grief. For families with deaf children, David Luterman has been a source for direction and comfort for more than 40 years. He describes strategies for coping with grief that I will briefly review here (Luterman, 2001).

Fight or Flight

In any stressful situation where fear, anxiety, anger, and other strong emotions are present, it is natural for people to do one of two things: run away from the situation or stay and deal with it. Flight or fight. When you first heard your child was deaf, you may have wanted to run away and hide. One father retreated alone to the family garage every time the stress got to be too much. His wife was left to deal with whatever was going on inside the house, alone. This is a normal and understandable response, but not a supportive one. Because you are reading this book, you are probably beyond dealing with the situation by denying it. However, your partner, spouse, other children, grandparents, and others may still be running away from the truth, at least occasionally. This is their way of coping. Talk about it with them as soon as you are able. Let them know you need their insights, strength, and courage, and when they are ready to face the truth, you'll be ready for their help and support. Let them know you need them in the present and focused on the current situation.

If there are other children in the family, pay particular attention. They, too, can use flight as a means of coping, but it may be harder for you to detect. Sometimes, it's impossible to separate normal childhood indifference from avoidance behaviors. Learning to cope is not easy or quick for kids either. Remember to be kind to yourself and others in your family, and they need to be kind to each other and you.

Did you know that a majority of couples with special needs children divorce? This is an extreme example of flight. Deafness in a child can be just as threatening to the stability of a family. You may already be experiencing problems with your partner. What you are going through may be normal, but that doesn't mean it can't be dangerous, especially if you are having trouble deciding what to do or if there is unresolved blame and guilt. This not only happens in weak marriages; it is possible in all marriages or relationships. One of our families reported having a very stable marriage and happy family life prior to their daughter losing her hearing at age 6 months. Within 12 months of the news, there was trouble in the family. The incredible amount of stress reported by both parents is withering: going through hearing aids, CI surgery, and subsequent speech therapy, along with making decisions about what to do and worrying about money. The marriage was dangerously close to ending. If there is this much risk in a relatively healthy marriage, imagine what can happen in one less than ideal? One parent who counsels other CI couples emphasizes the importance of hanging on and hanging together until a point of relief is reached. When the stress finally abates (and it does), you can "catch your breath." The catch-your-breath moment came for this parent counselor when, after 3 years post-implantation, her daughter had caught up developmentally to her chronological age. This mom's sound advice continues: your family needs to stay together; the grief and stress won't last forever; hold on tight all the way through to the other side. You will be glad you did.

You will not be overreacting if you seek professional counseling to help you through the process. Not being prepared for this possibility leaves you vulnerable for even greater stress and grief. Have the name of a marriage counselor, minister or rabbi, or other trusted professional ready in case you need help in coping with the deafness of your child.

Taking Control

Once the decision is made to face the situation, there may be a need to "take control." Luterman calls this *strategy modification*. The human need to change what is causing the family upheaval is understandable. If a child is sick, you care for him, take him to the doctor, cool his head with a moist cloth, change the linens, bring fresh flowers, read, and so on. You cope with the distress of the ill child by doing, by taking control. There is nothing wrong with this, is there? Be cautious, though. Some things can't be changed or controlled, and trying to do so can lead to disappointment and despair. The prayer of Reinhold Niebuhr, later adopted by Alcoholics Anonymous, speaks to this:

> . . . grant me the serenity
>
> to accept the things I cannot change;
>
> courage to change the things I can;
>
> and the wisdom to know the difference.

You can begin to take control by directing your energy to getting auditory stimulation (sound) to your child as soon as you can. If you choose a CI, you must get it done as soon as you possibly can. If you choose amplification with hearing aids, the same is true. Your child will have the best results the sooner he hears.

Reframing

If you accept that you can't change your child's deafness, you may cope with it by trying to think and speak of the situation in a new way. "Things could be worse." "Look on the bright side." "We'll get through this together; it will make us stronger." These phrases may or may not be helpful to you. But it is important to start thinking about deafness in ways other than negative. I asked one mother about letting go of expectations she had for her child and she emphatically responded, "I never let go of those expectations! I knew my daughter would be able to do anything she wanted, and my job was to give her that chance." Parents who are farther along than you are in the process can really help. Meet their deaf child(ren). See how they have developed into wonderful, loving children and how their parents love them. Don't get me wrong; deaf kids can be as obnoxious, rude, loud, and disrespectful as any other child. But that is exactly what you need to learn: your kid is going to be who he is; and he will be wonderful, warts and all.

Stress Reduction

Luterman's final coping strategy is learning to deal directly with your stress in order to reduce it. No two people do this in the same way. Some find comfort in walking or a good run. Some find golf or tennis or some other sporting activity a stress reducer. Music, cooking, aromatherapy, a full-body massage, or a simple hot bath may also bring soothing results. It is often suggested that keeping a journal of your thoughts, feelings, and progress has a calming, stress-reducing effect. Whatever it is, do it; take care of you.

Sometimes the stress reduction strategy is confused with the coping strategy of flight. Going to a movie or bowling when the rest of your family is meeting with the audiologist is not a healthy way to cope. It might relieve your stress, but it is, in truth, a means of escaping and doesn't help your stress in the long run. Meeting with the audiologist first, and then going to a movie together is a productive way to face the reality and reduce the stress. It's all right to do things for you; in fact, it is mandatory. Remember, the flight attendant always says, in case of emergency, place the oxygen mask on your face first before you give it to your child. It does the child no good if you are passed out from lack of air.

Recommendations for further reading are listed in the resources section of this book.

Questions to Ask Yourselves

As you and your family think about whether or not to pursue cochlear implantation, please consider these questions: Do you want your child to be part of the hearing and speaking world? How much time are you willing to dedicate to the CI process? What are the criteria for implantation? What is the process? Are you prepared for a less than perfect outcome? Finally, do you wonder if your family is strong enough to handle the difficulties of having a deaf child? One by one, let's look at these questions and what they mean.

Success with Hearing and Speaking

Whether you are deaf or hearing parents, you are reading this book because you are contemplating cochlear implantation and that means you are seeking something different from silence and sign language for your child—a different world from what he's in now. CIs have helped thousands of children experience sound. This, in turn, has helped them develop language and speech. The possibility of normal or near normal speech and language development is very real. I say *possibility* because there is wide variability of success with implanted children, and most of the causes for these differences remain unexplained. One child with an implant may develop speech that sounds no different from their normal hearing brother or sister, while another child with the same amount of loss and the same type implant and trained by the same teachers may have speech that does not sound entirely normal. Some children simply don't feel comfortable with the sounds the implant is making. Some children experience headaches, ringing, buzzing, and other unwanted noises and sensations and choose not to wear the implant. There is no clear explanation for this difference, and some researchers have dedicated themselves to finding out why there is so much variability.

Although a successful outcome can't be assumed before you decide on implantation, there are some general principles you need to know. Timing is important for success with CIs. The sooner the implant is turned on after the discovery of deafness, the sooner the brain is stimulated by sound. The earliest years in your child's life are the most important for language development. And, so, as a general rule, children implanted before the age of 2 or 3 years have better speech and language than children implanted when they are older.

Finding a Cochlear Implant Center

There are three ways to find a CI center that suits your family: referral from other families, referral from professionals, and finding centers through your own research.

Talk to Other Parents

Experienced parents are experts (as you soon will be) in the process of cochlear implantation. Only parents can tell you how they were treated as a family and whether the CI team lived up to its claims. Not all programs are created equal, but it is impossible to see that from the outside looking in. It can't be stressed enough how much assistance other families can offer you in finding the right CI center.

Talk with Professionals

Your primary care physician should make the appropriate referral to an otolaryngologist when hearing loss is suspected. In turn, the otolaryngologist should make a referral to the CI team, *if she knows of one.* In large metropolitan areas, this won't be a concern. In some geographical areas, where there are no large medical centers, not everyone (even professionals) knows of the closest, let alone the best, services available to you.

If your child is currently receiving services such as speech therapy or physical therapy, ask those providers for referral information. School districts also have information regarding services for families with deaf children and may be consulted even if you don't have a school-aged child.

Your Own Research

It's always a good idea to get a second opinion, and doing your own research can accomplish this. You can start looking for a program by contacting the three companies that make CIs approved by the federal Food and Drug Administration, the FDA. You can contact them by phone, toll free, or by visiting their Web sites (contact information is in the resources section of this book). These companies have clinic and program information for locations all over the world. Each company has representatives working with every CI program who can give you specific answers to your questions about the services each CI program offers. Once you have names and locations of CI programs, you can phone the center directly and make arrangements to visit. It is an extremely good idea to meet at least some of the CI professionals at the center or program (not all programs are located in one building, but in several offices at different locations) to see if it is the right place for you. We suggest you determine if the center's philosophy is that of putting the family, not just the child, at the center of the process. You, as parent, are the constant in your child's life as well as the support system and the decision maker. You should be at the center of the CI team assigned to work with you (Jerger et al., 2001). If you don't get this feeling when visiting or talking to a CI program, consider going elsewhere.

Qualifications for Implantation

Your child must meet certain criteria to be a candidate for cochlear implantation. Figure 1–1 shows there are five basic conditions that must be present for you to be on track for an implant. Determining these five basics is the first thing a CI team will do. Your child must have a sensorineural hearing loss in both ears, receive no meaningful help from hearing aids, and show no progress in hearing or listening skills. These evaluations include a medical examination of the ear to make sure there are no abnormalities or infections that would rule out surgery. Hearing tests determine your child's level of hearing loss and attempt to measure what, if any, benefit is received from hearing aids. Speech and language testing, when appropriate, will determine a baseline development marker to be used to measure future progress. With infants and very young children, you will be asked to report your observations of your child's babbling or speaking as well as listening behavior. There will also be some sort of imaging testing with computerized tomography (CAT or CT scan) or a magnetic resonance image (MRI) test to determine the suitability of the inner ear and auditory nerve for implantation and which cochlea might be better to

---

To be considered for an implant your child must:

- Have severe to profound hearing loss in both ears
- Receive limited or no benefit from hearing aids
- Have a family that is committed to helping the child learn how to hear
- Have a family with realistic expectations
- Be healthy enough to have surgery including all middle ear health issues resolved

---

Figure 1–1. Criteria for cochlear implant candidacy.

implant. As needed, there may also be referrals for physical therapy, occupational therapy, and psychological evaluations.

The final criterion for implantation may be surprising, but perhaps the most important: the entire family must be highly motivated to achieve success and must have realistic expectations for the outcome. Like having a soccer star or a dancer in the family, many activities will revolve around your deaf child, the process of getting an implant, and caring for it afterward. Appointments with the speech pathologist for A-V sessions and with the audiologist for adjustments to the implant, batteries, cords, and other pieces of equipment will constantly be part of the plans. As your child gets older, most of this responsibility can be his and becomes less central to family life. But you've got to get that far along for the payoff!

The Cochlear Implant Process

If your child meets the qualifying criteria and you decide to proceed with an implant, the next steps can be seen in Figure 1-2. You, with the advice of the CI team, will select which device to implant, the surgeon's office schedules surgery, the surgery occurs, and the initial stimulation happens about 1 week after surgery; then you attend regularly scheduled sessions with your audiologist for adjustments and training. If speech therapy is initiated, it will continue post-implantation. After the first year, visits to the audiologist should occur at least annually to ensure the implant is working properly and to make any needed adjustments. Other therapies will continue as needed. Following chapters discuss this process in more detail.

Making the Decision

It wasn't so long ago that the average age of a child brought in for hearing evaluation due to parental concern was 18 months. Even though hearing loss is one of the most common birth deficiencies in the United States, babies were not screened for it before they left the hospital until recently. Parents didn't know whether their child could hear or not. Families generally assume that the baby's hearing is just fine, especially with all that crying going on. Several months pass and somebody starts to notice that things aren't quite right. Perhaps the

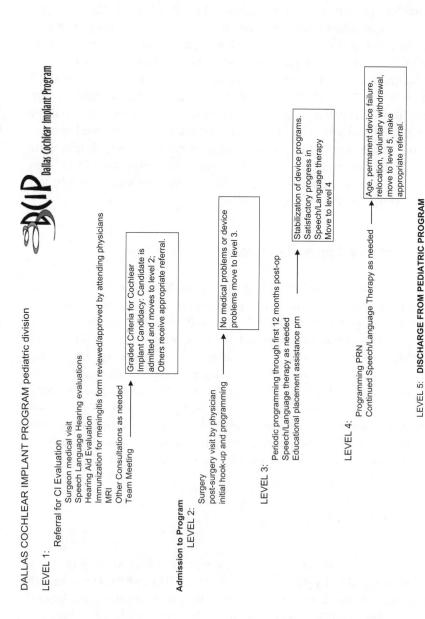

Figure 1–2. This flowchart shows a typical progression through a pediatric CI program from initial referral to discharge.

12

mom or dad or a grandparent starts paying particular attention to the infant's hearing and notices there is no response to loud noise or soft sounds that are close enough to hear. Other family members may deny this and make excuses. Months go by, more observations of unusual behavior occur, and finally, the truth can't be denied: something is wrong with the baby's hearing. This may have been your experience. If so, compare it with those parents who learned of their child's potential hearing loss before they left the hospital because of a failed hearing screening test performed shortly (hours!) after birth. Rather than a gradual shift from denial to action, the parents are immediately faced with a hard, bittersweet reality: their baby is here but deaf (and perhaps with other impairments and concerns, too). Gathering strength over time to face deafness and develop a plan of action sounds good; but now, before you've even taken your child home, the struggle begins. Not only are you deprived of at least a few months of not being concerned with hearing loss; now you are told you must make a decision about what to do as soon as possible.

What Is Right?

Loving, reasonable parents want what is best for their children. You want to do the right thing, but what is it? Although the good news is there are people there ready to advise you, the more difficult news is that the ultimate choice is up to you, and you need to make it as soon as you can. Why the hurry? Your baby's brain is growing rapidly now and sound needs to be part of that growth for language development. There will be more on this later.

In your research, you will find an abundance of competing information in books and articles, on the Internet, and from CI specialists, hearing aid specialists, and the Deaf community about what each thinks is best for your deaf child. Some of the issues where conflict arises are the concerns for Deaf culture, disability versus trait, informed consent and autonomy (making decisions on behalf of minors), and whether the future will be open or limited.

Deaf Culture

In talking about the deaf community, I am relying on two respected organizations, The Alexander Graham Bell Association for Deaf and

Hard of Hearing (AG Bell) and the National Association of the Deaf (NAD) to inform the discussion. The Deaf community (capital *D* to distinguish the group's use of American Sign Language) in the United States, a culture rich with tradition, history, and customs, is made up of a diverse group of people, usually born deaf, and their families whose primary mode of communication is American Sign Language (ASL). Deaf persons who speak (are oral) and hearing persons who sign are minority members of the community due to the understandably important role ASL has to the culture. There is a network of Deaf communities across the country usually close to deaf educational opportunities.

Approximately 90% of deaf children are born to hearing parents. Therefore, the growth of the Deaf community depends on new members who come from the hearing world. The concern among the community is understandable: will CIs for infants and children diminish future membership in the Deaf community?

The NAD position statement on CIs reminds us that the medical-surgical model of deafness is only one viewpoint. There exists another model: the wellness model. While the medical-surgical model considers deafness a disability and an abnormality needing to be fixed, the NAD's wellness model considers deafness to be a normal human trait. The statement maintains that deafness, accordingly, does not keep people from living whole and complete lives, from being psychologically and emotionally strong, or from contributing to the community at large. Nor does deafness need to be fixed.

In the early days of implantation, the Deaf community thought it barbaric to perform "unnecessary" surgery in order to alter a non-life-threatening trait. Position statements from Deaf organizations, including the NAD, showed clear and strong reservations about the CI process, citing its elective, potentially dangerous nature and limited success with the first implantees. (Incidentally, we now know that the limited success of early recipients was due to implant candidacy criteria being too broad; people were implanted who had limited potential for benefit for various reasons having nothing to do with the device per se.) While the NAD position on implants has softened over time, the Deaf community is still reluctant to embrace cochlear implantation without reservations. They rightly claim that implants don't cure deafness and that not all outcomes are predictable or successful. They call for more research to determine if the risks of implantation are worth the proven benefits.

The AG Bell organization has a different approach from the NAD's wellness model and advocates for the deaf "to listen, talk and thrive in mainstream society" (AG Bell, 2008). The organization has always been a supporter of oral education and using technologies, including hearing aids and CIs, to that end. The importance of spoken language and the necessity of hearing the nuances of language are part of the philosophy of AG Bell. If language defines reality, as the linguist de Saussure stated (Saussure, 1916), then unlimited language development means unlimited reality, a broadening rather than a narrowing of possibilities.

Scientific research conducted since 1991 (the first year of FDA approval for the multichannel implant) has indeed shown that successful outcomes for children with CIs are a reasonable expectation. What is a successful outcome? Some indicators of success include that appropriately implanted children are catching up to their typical hearing peers in language and speech development within a few years of implantation, that they are enrolled in regular classrooms and have hearing and deaf friends, and that they experience high user satisfaction (see Chapters 2 and 10). Once a young child has been implanted, the rate of speech and language learning is similar to normal hearing children.

Our program, the Dallas Cochlear Implant Program, approaches CI with the bias that it is better to hear than not and that parents alone have the right to make this decision on behalf of their child.

All things considered, we believe the possible benefits of cochlear implantation outweigh any potential risks.

Informed Consent and Autonomy

Another contentious issue, not only in the Deaf community, but with biomedical ethicists in general, is that of informed consent and autonomy. Informed consent is defined as the process of being thoroughly informed about a project (in this case, receiving a CI) and your participation in it including all the risks and benefits. Autonomy means that individuals have the right to make informed decisions on their own behalf (for themselves). Put another way, no one has the right to make someone else participate in a procedure in which he doesn't want to participate. All medical procedures require an informed consent of some kind demonstrating that we agree to participate and assume the risks involved. Parents do this on behalf of their children in all life-threatening situations, but CI is not life threatening. Why not wait until the child is old enough to make the decision himself?

Research done in our program, as well as many other research institutions, has demonstrated time and again that if a child was deafened before he started developing language (prelingual), there is a window of opportunity of about 3 years to maximize his positive hearing outcome. This is due to the way the brain develops in infants and young children. That development is rapid through the first 3 years of life and probably hits its high point about age 6. To be implanted before age 3 is best, and as soon as possible after discovery of deafness is ideal. It has been demonstrated repeatedly that the hearing part of the deaf child's brain can "catch up" with normal hearing children faster and more definitively the sooner the implant is received and certainly before age 3. The longer the child waits for auditory stimulation, the steeper the mountain for speech perception, speech production, and language to develop normally. Your CI team should be able to bring to focus realistic expectations based on your child's unique case.

Further, there are some medical circumstances that require an even faster decision. If your child has had meningitis, the bony structure of the inner ear (cochlea) is at risk for thickening due to bony growth called ossification. Eventually, this thickening can block the chamber where the implant is supposed to go. Once that happens (and it can happen rapidly), the chances of successful implantation diminish greatly. Any situation causing this ossification is reason enough for a quick decision. This is literally a matter of days and weeks, not months and years.

According to Joel Feinberg (Feinberg, 1980), children's rights can be divided into four categories: rights that children and adults hold in common; rights that only children have; rights that only adults have; and rights in trust (rights that are to be saved until the child is an adult). Autonomy and the right to informed consent is a right you hold in trust for your child. Your decision not to implant would take these two rights away. How? Your child will be deaf whether or not he receives an implant. Should she want to become a member of the Deaf community when she grows up, there will be nothing stopping her from it. But if the child grows up wanting to be a speaking person participating in the hearing world, the decision to delay implantation will have made the right to decide moot. There will be no need for informed consent because there is no autonomy. Be mindful of what Harvey Cox

(1967) said, "Not to decide is to decide." Your decision has the opportunity to limit the choices of your child or to provide what Feinberg calls an open future, a future that holds the most options and opportunities in which the rights you were entrusted with are preserved.

Final Thoughts

What is best for a deaf child in a hearing world?

You've heard conflicting information about cochlear implantation. There are many sides to the discussion as to whether implantation is a wise decision for your child. There are those who feel that your child should make his own decision so it is best to wait until he is old enough to understand what is at stake. Many in the Deaf community don't agree that hearing and speaking are necessary for a high quality life and that implantation for that purpose is cruel and unusual. Some people feel it is unethical to give proxy consent to a life-changing surgical procedure for something not life threatening.

Your job is this: you need to make a decision about your baby's mode of communication: will it be hearing and speaking, signing, or both? If hearing and speaking is your choice, you need to make the decision as soon as you can. You need to find other families who have deaf children. You need to find a CI center that suits you. You're going to commit your entire family for the rest of your lives to this project. All of this must be taken into consideration when you are making your choice. This is quite a challenge, so get all the help and support you can. Remember, you are not alone.

Reference List

AG Bell. (2008). Retrieved October 15, 2008, from http://www.agbell.org/D esktopDefault.aspx?p=Who We Are

Bristor, M. (1984). The birth of a handicapped child—A holistic model for grieving. *Family Relations, 33,* 25-32.

Clark, J. G. & English, K. M. (2004). *Counseling in audiological practice: helping patients and families adjust to hearing loss.* Upper Saddle River, NJ: Pearson.

Cox, H. G. (1967). *On not leaving it to the snake* (p. viii). New York: Macmillan.

Feinberg, J. (1980). The child's right to an open future. In W. Aiken & H. LaFollette (Eds.), *Whose child? Children's rights, parental authority, and state power* (pp. 124–153). Totowa, NJ: Littlefield, Adams & Co.

Jerger, S., Roeser, R., & Tobey, E. (2001). Management of hearing loss in infants: The UTD/Callier Center Position Statement. *Journal of the American Academy of Audiology, 12*, 329–336.

Kubler-Ross, E. (1969). *On death and dying.* New York: Macmillian.

Luterman, D. (2001). *Counseling persons with communication disorders and their families* (4th ed.). Austin, TX: Pro-Ed.

Saussure, F. D. (1916). *Course in general linguistics.* London: Fontana/Collins.

Chapter 2

Will My Child Learn to Talk?

By Emily A. Tobey

Stop. Stop right now. Listen. What do you hear? Do you hear your heart racing, your breath rapidly going in and out? Do you hear the traffic, birds singing, water running through a creek, the hum from lights, or the low pulsing of a loud radio played by a bunch of teenagers? Do you hear the airplanes overhead? Listen, carefully. Now, take a moment and imagine. Imagine a quiet world. Imagine the world your child will experience.

Listening is integral to speaking. When hearing is stopped, as in deafness, or muted, as in hearing losses, learning to speak is a difficult task requiring intensive, directed training focusing on the correct placement to produce sounds, feeling how air is directed through those structures, and working in small steps to build sounds into words and words into sentences. This is a difficult task that many teachers and deaf children engage in during the development of communication.

As you will learn in other places in this book, cochlear implants (CIs) do not completely restore hearing, but for many children, the signal generated by the implant provides enough information to develop spoken communication. This electrical signal provides important feedback to your child that allows her to adjust and expand early sounds into words and sentences as she learns to associate what she hears with what she says.

Modes of Communication and Why Listening Is Important for Learning to Speak

One of the first decisions your family makes when you learn your child is deaf relates to how you will communicate as a family and as individuals interacting with your child. We refer to these methods of communicating as *modes of communication*. Many families will opt to communicate by listening and talking only, because nearly 90% of deaf children are born to hearing parents. Other families may elect to incorporate hand and finger signs representing words or letters into their communication but follow the grammar rules of their spoken language. Yet other families may elect to communicate with two languages or more than two languages. Modes of communication sometimes change over time to reflect the evolving needs of your family, your child, and the communities your child interacts with on a daily basis.

Communication refers to the common system of spoken words, signs, symbols, or behaviors used to tell someone what you are thinking about. The most common ways of communicating include talking, listening, writing, reading, or gesturing. Modes of communication refer to the range of mechanisms available for your family to do this within a given language. For example, you might communicate using an auditory-oral mode of communication (listening + speaking) or a total communication mode of communication (listening + speaking + signing). These modes of communication are typically based on a language (English, French, and Japanese); thus, you might learn the spoken words and signs depicting the words of these languages. American Sign Language (ASL), on the other hand, represents a systematic language rich in its complexity of vocabulary and grammar. It is not a simple translation of spoken English into signs. It differs in many important ways from spoken English or English conveyed by signs such as in Signing Exact English (SEE). Rather than conveying an idea via a word and grammar derived from English, ASL conveys ideas with a different vocabulary and word order. ASL also differs from French Sign Language (*Langue des signes française*, or LSF), German Sign Language (*Deutsche Gebär-densprache*, or DSL), or any other sign language in ways as significant as spoken English differs from spoken French, German, Vietnamese. Introducing ASL means you and your family will need to learn a foreign language, just as though you were going to learn Spanish if you were a native English speaker. Thus, your family needs to decide what language you will introduce to your child and how you will do it.

Listening provides important information about the world around you. You gain important information about your safety by listening to the sounds in your environment that alert you to danger. You gain internal pleasure by listening to your favorite radio station. You also gain important information about how to interpret a message by listening to the melody of people's speech. Are they asking a question? Are they excited? Is something wrong? Are they making a subtle joke? Listening allows your child to hear his own speech, as well as the speech of other people around him (Figure 2-1). Your child will learn to listen to his own voice and to experiment with how to match his speech to your community. All children will engage in verbal play. Your child will explore his mouth, hands, and feet. Babies like to put things in their mouths, they like to blow bubbles, and they like to feel their fingers and toes. Your job is to encourage your baby to play and explore—all, of course, when you know it is safe to do so.

Under most circumstances, you and I always hear something. If we are put into a totally quiet situation, we alert and begin to pay special attention to our environment. Our brain puts us on alert for possible danger and tells us to be careful—to pay attention carefully to what is around us. We learn that sound can warn us of danger. We

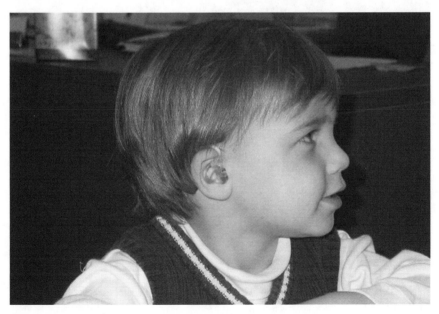

Figure 2–1. John is listening intently to his mother.

tend to sit quietly and look around our environment a lot. Our eyes gaze around and we watch carefully.

Deaf children also watch their environment. They carefully look around to find what activity concerns them. The initial sounds from a CI are startling, new, and scary. It is okay. Even hearing babies, when learning to listen, are startled and scared by unfamiliar, loud sounds in their environment. As your child adjusts to a CI, he will learn that sound is an important tool for telling him when he is in danger, when he needs to pay attention, and when he wants to learn about activities in the environment. It is important that your child wear the CI as much as possible. Children who wear their implants consistently, all day long, are better communicators than children who wear their implants only part of the day (Figure 2-2).

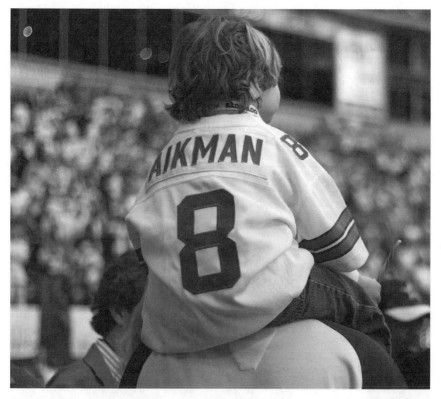

Figure 2–2. Ben is attending a night football game wearing his implant.

Will My Child Learn to Talk?

The simplest answer is yes, your child will learn to talk—but I will add to this that you, as a parent, play a major role in how well your child learns to talk. It is important for you to love your child by touching, hugging, kissing, and encouraging your child to watch you and imitate you. You provide an important model for your child while she learns to talk and interact with the world around her. Deaf children who become good talkers come from families that love them and include them in all family activities. Good talkers come from homes where they are an integral part of family life. Good talkers come from homes that expect their children to talk and to talk well. Good talkers come from homes that adopt a consistent signal (like a questioning body shrug) to tell a CI child it is time to listen or to talk.

Before CIs, young children with a severe-to-profound sensorineural hearing loss using conventional high-powered hearing aids were understood by other listeners only about 20% of the time when they spoke. As the technology for CIs improves, children using CIs are understood by larger numbers of listeners and by listeners who are unfamiliar with listening to deaf children talk.

Many studies show deaf children using CIs are understood 50 to 80% of the time by listeners. Children who use CIs must develop several communication skills at the same time in order to be successful at getting their message across to others when talking. These talking skills include pronouncing the sounds of their native language, putting sounds together to form words, building a vocabulary that allows them to express their ideas, and developing a grammar that orders the words into a message a listener understands.

In the Beginning Months

During most of the first year of life, deaf and hearing babies sound alike. Many parents who do not learn their child is deaf in the hospital at birth may not know their child is deaf because of this fact. Babies are immature in their brain and body. The baby must mature in order to begin the steps involved in communication.

During the early months of the first year of life, all babies in all cultures generate similar sounds. Young babies cry, squeal, growl, produce raspberries, and form vowel- or consonant-like sounds. In the early months of life, the brain begins to build connections within itself and to other structures in the head, body, arms, and legs. As these connections form, the head begins to grow away from the body forming a neck, the tongue and jaw begin to act independently of one another, and the limbs begin to strengthen, allowing your baby to eat semisolid foods, roll over, sit, and crawl. During these early formative stages, all babies are capable of producing the sounds generated in any language. Even at about 2 or 3 months of age, your baby will try to imitate the mouth movements you make. She will try to smile, stick out her tongue, and purse her lips to try to blow.

Around 8 to 10 months of age, hearing babies begin to babble producing combinations of vowel and consonant sounds. It is during these early babbling days that deaf babies begin to behave differently than hearing babies. Young hearing babies form their first syllables by producing the vowels and consonants of their native language—they play to themselves making speech sounds (Figure 2–3). Syllables are

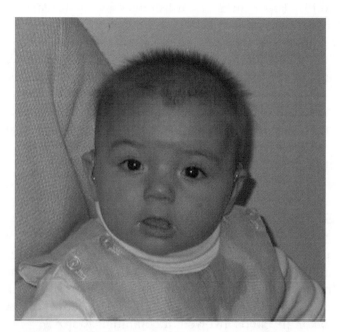

Figure 2–3. Todd is vocalizing and paying close attention to the speaker.

important because they form one of the critical building blocks for saying words. Deaf babies often continue to produce the simple vocalizations associated with squealing, growling, crying, and raspberries. Deaf babies may remain in the earliest vocalization stage until they are 3 or 4 years or older.

You will be encouraged to provide your baby with hearing aids or CIs at the earliest possible time in order to make sure that your baby has the best possible hearing; this will help your baby make the transition from early vocalizations to these early syllables. Even a little bit of hearing goes a long way in helping your baby move into this second babbling stage.

What else should you expect? Deaf and hearing babies engage in "intentional" communication attempts between 8 and 12 months of age. Your baby will want to "talk" and get you to pay attention to her. Hearing and deaf babies make eye contact with you; they use gestures consistently (opening and closing the hand when they want something) to gain your attention. Hearing and deaf babies try over and over to gain your attention when they are not understood. Two of the best predictors of how well your deaf baby will learn to talk after receiving a CI are how often she tries to gain your attention when she wants to tell you about something and how often she starts a communication with you, rather than simply following your lead when you want to tell her something. As your deaf baby gets used to hearing sound from a hearing aid or a CI, she will use gestures and vocalizations to try to communicate with you. You need to be patient and try to respond to her as often as possible in order to encourage her to continue trying to communicate.

In these very earliest communications, it is normal to use gestures and speech with a young baby or toddler. It is important for you to play and to talk with your baby. Typical parents talk to their babies in "baby talk." Although many parents claim they do not use baby talk with their baby, close study indicates parents adjust their speaking style when talking with young babies. Typical parents raise their pitch higher and exaggerate the melody of their sentences. Typical parents often pair their exaggerated speech with exaggerated gestures to illustrate their points. For example, you may take your child's hand and wave it while saying, "Say bye-bye," when you finish a conversation or when you are leaving a situation with other people. By pairing the use of the gesture and the word *bye-bye*, you provide a consistent model of how communication is ended in many situations. The combined use of a gesture and appropriate vocabulary also encourages other people who are around your baby to interact and communicate with her. Another example of how parents adjust their speech when talking with their baby lies in the choice of vocabulary they use.

You also may unconsciously adjust your level of vocabulary by using words like *potty* or using sounds to indicate words, like *moooo* for a cow, or *choo-choo* for a train. It is normal to use parental baby talk to let your child know you are paying attention to her and you are willing to talk with her. As a parent, you model communication to your baby by talking and explaining. For example, you may change your baby's diaper. Suddenly, like a flash of brilliant sunlight, your baby smiles at you. Unconsciously, typical parents begin talking to their babies, saying, "What a sweet smile. You look so sweet. Yes, that's a real sweet smile. Oh, tickle, tickle. Let me see that sweet smile again." Parents model speech and encourage their babies to interact with them and engage in communication.

During these early communication times, you will encourage your baby to interact and learn. You might do this in a game with a stuffed animal, such as a cat, by saying, "Look, what is this? It is a cat. Meow. The cat says meow." You will play games with your baby to let your baby learn what a routine is. For example, you may lift your baby up to the sky and say, "Whew. Here we go flying," and then pause waiting for your baby to smile and indicate she wants more. You will repeat the game over and over, thus training your child to have fun with you. These early interactions of playing with your baby help her learn that communication and sharing are fun.

Deaf and hearing babies respond to these interactive communications. You should build as many of these opportunities for early communication as you can into your child's routine. Your child learns through these repetitive games and interactions that you are willing to communicate with him and that you expect him to communicate to the best of his abilities with you. These games and interactions should be times of intense pleasure and enjoyment. By showing your love to your child, you model how much fun spoken communication is. Children who use CIs become good talkers when their families spend time talking with them and encourage them to interact with others.

Deaf children who use CIs follow many of these early steps of beginning to vocalize and babble as soon as they are implanted. In many cases, deaf children using CIs will move from one stage to another stage of talking very rapidly over a few months. The first 6 months of listening with a CI is a very important time, with some of the biggest and fastest changes in talking occurring during this time. Even though you may feel overwhelmed with learning how to take care of the CI, how to change batteries, how to encourage your baby to wear it, it is important that you encourage your baby to wear the implant during all waking hours. It is important that you spend time loving and playing and talking with your child during this early period so your child will learn how much fun it is to communicate by listening and talking.

What Happens Next?

Talking involves the pattern of sounds our mouths generate in our language. Talking also includes the construction of words and the units needed to change meanings of words. Talking requires a child to learn how to combine simple words to form more complex words. Talking necessitates the correct ordering of words in a grammar and using the words appropriately in a variety of social contexts. Talking in young children requires maturation of the brain; maturation of the structures of the lungs, head, and ear; *and* social interactions with people in their environment (Figure 2–4).

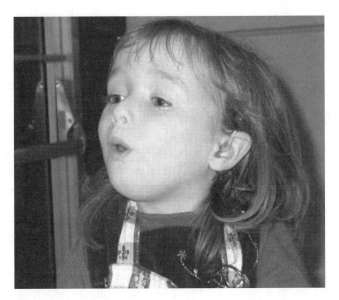

Figure 2–4. Megan is practicing an *oooooo* sound.

During talking, the primary sounds are conveyed by vowels and consonants. Vowels are relatively simple to make by rather gross adjustments to the opening of the jaw and placement of the tongue in the mouth. These movement patterns produce sounds that are relatively loud, long in duration, and relatively low in pitch. Vowels are some of the first sounds acquired by hearing babies. Deaf babies also say vowels but usually only a limited set produced by relatively simple openings of the jaw and tongue. Deaf children using CIs find vowels easiest to say correctly.

Consonants require precise coordination of the muscles in the larynx and mouth. Consonants occur rapidly, sometimes within a few thousandths of a second. Consonants are softer than vowels, shorter in duration, and composed of higher pitches. The combination of soft loudness, higher pitches, and shorter durations makes consonants hard to master, even for many hearing children, and even harder to master for children who do not hear. In many hearing children, consonants are not fully mastered until the elementary school ages.

It is not unusual for you and your family to understand what your child is saying when people who do not know your child may not. This is a common occurrence for normal hearing children. I still remember babysitting my grandson when he was around 4. He would sit on my lap talking and telling me about everything he was interested in. I nodded my head and continued to say, "Really, tell me more about it," although I had no clue what he was excited about telling me. Finally, my daughter, while laughing, would say, "Grand Em, David is telling you about Pokemon people." Your child needs to learn to talk to family members and to talk to other people outside the family. As a parent, you need to encourage your child to talk with family members and with others outside the family. Help your child communicate by helping other people learn to understand what your child is saying.

Vowels and consonants form the building blocks for developing syllables, words, phrases, and sentences. Consonants are particularly important because they convey information about the message that allows a listener to fill in the blanks by using situational or contextual cues. One of the easiest ways to understand the differing roles of consonants and vowels is to watch the television program, "Wheel of Fortune." On this program, people win money for accurately guessing consonants and pay out money to "buy" vowels. The "win-buy" situation works because many people can accurately guess a message from just the consonants. Children practice this skill in many childhood games including Hangman. In this game, children think of a word, recall the sounds in the words, and write down an underscore for each sound in the word. Other children guess what sounds are the underscores. If they guess wrong, the score is recorded as a drawn segment of the man hanging. The best players at Hangman guess consonants first and typically learn, from trial and error, the consonant sounds that occur most often and least often in their language. They learn to guess vowels last.

By listening with a CI, your child learns the sound patterns of her language. The pattern of consonant and vowel combinations that form syllables and words is language dependent. For example, 24 different consonants are used in spoken English, but only eight consonants are used in the native language of Hawaiian. When your child hears, she learns the rules of how sounds are combined and the patterns of combination that are acceptable for her language. When your child hears and learns the sound patterns associated with the language, she also learns to say the sounds. Your child will make mistakes in ordering and correctly pronouncing sounds—all children make mistakes while they are in the learning stage. Your job is to encourage your child to listen and talk and gently guide pronunciations to match your model.

It is important to encourage your child to listen and watch other people when they are talking with your child. Very small changes in mouth positions result in different consonants. You experience these differences when you say, "see" or "she." Look in a mirror when you say "see." Notice your lips smile. Notice when you say "she" your lips round as if you kiss the air. Listen to the pitch of the sounds: "see, she." The overall pitch of *see* is higher than *she*. Just a slight change in your lip positions makes the difference. As you encourage your child to attend to the faces and speech of other speakers, your child will build a model of how to say consonants and vowels correctly.

Consonants form the beginning or end of many syllables. Examples of words beginning and ending with consonants include *hot*, *dog*, *pop*, *corn*. When syllables are combined to form complex words, consonants appear in the beginning, middle, and end of words. Examples of more complex words include *hot dog* and *popcorn*. Many early word combinations have the consonant at the beginning and middle of the words. For example, *ma* and *me* combine to form *mommy*. Deaf children hear consonants in the beginning of words more accurately than they hear consonants in the middle or end of words. CIs help children hear consonants in all positions of words; however, your child may need extra encouragement to "tune" into the consonants at the middle and end of words. The sounds at the end of words are very important and a deaf child who fails to say them will fail to communicate important concepts like time (*walks*—present tense; *walked*—past tense) or quantity (*duck*—one; *ducks*—more than one).

Deaf children who use CIs are able to pronounce vowels and consonants more correctly than deaf children who use hearing aids. Deaf children who use CIs also are able to correctly pronounce sounds in complex words made up of more than one syllable. More importantly, deaf children who use CIs are able to produce sounds in the final position of words more accurately than deaf children who use hearing aids. Deaf children who use CIs also learn the melody of sentences more accurately than deaf children who use hearing aids. Your child will learn to understand when you are asking a question, when you are excited, when you are setting a boundary by saying "no," and when you have finished a sentence and want him to respond. Each of these simple communication situations is signaled by a change in the melody of your voice through changes in your pitch and duration. Your child will learn the rules and meanings of these melody changes and use them in his own talking. Your child will become a good talker as he learns to listen with his CI and as he learns to say sounds in all parts of a word and change the melody of his talking. You are your child's best cheerleader, so help your child learn to say these sounds and adjust the melodies to say sentences or questions. It is important to tell your child how well he is doing over and over.

The Vocabulary Explosion

As your child learns sounds and puts them into words, her vocabulary grows. A typically developing child starts learning a new word every week, and then the child learns a new word every day. By about 4 or 5 years of age, typical children learn a new word every 2 hours they are awake. Many typically developing children will have a vocabulary of around 5000 words by the time they are in kindergarten or first grade. Your child learns more vocabulary in the first 5 years of age then she learns in any other time period of her life. When your child is implanted, you want to help her catch up and increase her vocabulary.

This is a miraculous time and you help your child learn new vocabulary by reading books, playing games, and talking with her. Deaf children who use CIs develop larger vocabularies than deaf children who use hearing aids. You help your child learn new vocabulary by reading and playing with her over and over. It is important to make time in your day to read to your child and to let your child tell the story back to you. Introduce new words to your child and let her repeat them back to you.

As your child learns more vocabulary, she learns to string together words to form simple sentences. Typically developing children say two-word sentences when they are 2 years old and three-word sentences when they are 3 years old. When your child is very young, she may say, "Boy fall," as a way to tell you about something she sees. "Boy fall" might mean "I sit down" or "My brother John tripped and fell" or "The boy who lives next door fell on the ball when it was hit into center field." Deaf children who use CIs learn to use longer and more complex sentences than deaf children who use hearing aids. You help your child learn to use longer and more complex sentences when you encourage your child to talk with you.

Your child strings together word combinations he is familiar with in order to describe new ideas he is experiencing. One of my favorite examples of a novel, two-word sentence comes from my friend, Andrea, who has very active twins. Andrea, who is in the hall listening to her daughter playing in another room, hears her daughter say, "Uh-oh boom," just before Andrea hears a crash and bang of toys.

Deaf children who use CIs develop longer memory spans than deaf children who use hearing aids, which helps them learn to say longer and longer sentences. As your child learns more vocabulary, he says a wider variety of sentences and longer sentences. Your child will learn to use context to understand the meaning of an ambiguous sentence such as, "The duck is ready to eat," which may indicate "The yellow duck outside by the pond is hungry and it is dinnertime" or the "The roasted duck, which mother cooked for 3 hours, is ready to be served for dinner." Children who use CIs are more accurate at determining the underlying meaning of sentences than deaf children who use hearing aids. Your child will learn to use the context of different situations to help understand messages and compose appropriate answers.

Your child also learns how to use language in different social situations: what to say at home, what to say in church, what to say in school. She learns to take turns talking and how to keep on a topic rather than changing topics. She learns how to communicate in difficult situations such as talking on the telephone to her grandparents or talking to her parents in a room full of people.

School and Educational Influences

Going to school is an important activity for your child when he is learning to talk, read, and write. School allows your child to interact with other children his own age. It is important for your child to interact with other children because children communicate with one another in a different way than when adults talk with children. Young children talking with their friends learn how to disagree, form friendships, and develop humor. Learning to talk with children their own age is an important skill that contributes to children being "good" talkers (Figure 2–5).

During preschool and kindergarten, your child is introduced to a variety of socially acceptable behaviors. Your child learns to wait his turn to talk and not to interrupt when another person is talking. Your child learns to sit quietly and to concentrate on one topic for a period of time. Your child learns how to make friends. As your child learns to talk with other children, he begins to play with his speech. Young children make up words (we typically call these words slang) or alter-

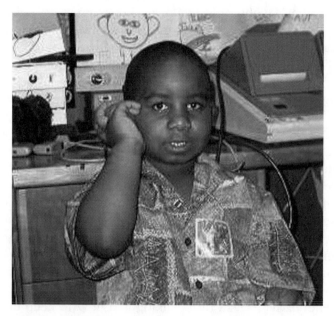

Figure 2–5. Scooter at school listening with his implant.

native meanings for words (when the word *bad* means "good"). Typically developing children enjoy making jokes and playing riddles. These word games rely on the sounds and meanings of words. Deaf children who use hearing aids often are unable to fully appreciate riddles because they miss some of the play on words. Children who use CIs learn to understand riddles because their improved listening with the CI helps them learn the play on words. When your child wears the implant consistently, he is exposed to these word games and learns to use these games in his own communication. Interactions with other children help your child learn to tell jokes and understand the jokes other children play.

As your child enters elementary school, she begins to understand that words are made up of sounds and that sounds are written with letters. Many young children first learn to associate spoken and printed words with logos through familiar activities. For example, many children will say "McDonald's" when they see the golden arches because they experienced getting a Happy Meal at McDonald's. Many classroom activities are designed to help your child learn to sound out words and to learn the letters of the alphabet. These activities form the beginning steps for learning to read.

Reading is a difficult process, but a very important process for your child to learn. Deaf children who rely on sign language to communicate often graduate from high school reading only at the second or third grade level. Deaf children who use CIs typically read at higher grade levels, and many deaf children using CIs read as well as hearing children of the same ages. Approximately 70% of children using CIs demonstrate reading comprehension levels at junior high or high school levels. A typical newspaper is written at about a sixth grade reading level, and recent reports suggest a person needs to read at a high school level to understand most of the information on the Internet. You will not want your child to miss out on this important information.

It is important for you to encourage your child to practice communicating by listening, speaking, reading, and writing. The elementary school years are spent learning *how* to read, whereas the middle and high school years are spent using reading to *learn new* information. Both of these activities are important for deaf children who use CIs. Deaf children with CIs perform higher on school tests examining how much knowledge they learn in a class than deaf children who do not have CIs.

Deaf children who experience time in a classroom with normal hearing children perform higher on school tests than deaf children who only spend time in special education classrooms. It is important to encourage your child in learning to read and learning new information. Setting consistent times to complete homework and to concentrate on learning new material assists your child in improving academic performance.

Will My Child Learn to Talk?

As I said at the beginning of this chapter, the simple answer is yes. The harder question to answer is, "How *well* will my child talk?" Several key factors are important for determining how well your child will talk. First, it is important to provide hearing aids or CIs as soon as possible so your child can begin the journey of learning to communicate. Second, it is important for your family to interact and talk with your cochlear implanted child to help her learn how to talk. Third, it is important to provide a consistent mode of communication that provides consistent listening and talking experiences. Fourth, your child may benefit from speech therapy services helping her learn to listen and talk. Fifth, encourage your child to play and interact with other children so your child enhances her communication experiences. Sixth, help your child develop an interest in reading by including a time for reading stories daily.

Learning to listen and talk is a personal journey your child will undertake. Your child's journey will be helped by your active and caring participation.

Emma's Story

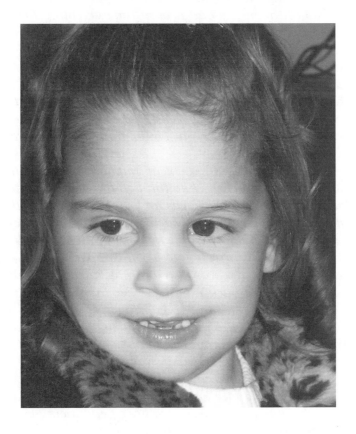

At birth, Emma passed her OAE newborn hearing screen before we were discharged from the hospital. She seemed like any other newborn responding to our voice and sounds around her. She began to say words like "mamma" and "dada" around her first birthday. But over the following months we noticed deterioration in Emma's speech.

As a few more months went by, we noticed that Emma was not developing speech. Our pediatrician recommended further evaluation with a local ENT. In November 2003, Emma was referred for an auditory brainstem response (ABR). We will never forget the morning of the ABR. We were shocked to learn that our daughter had a bilateral severe to profound sensorineural hearing loss. We immediately questioned the results and accuracy of the ABR. This led to a second objective opinion that arrived at the same exact conclusions. Even then, we had a hard time accepting the results. We searched for any way possible to prove that the tests may be inaccurate. We spent numerous hours researching medical journals and publications at the University of Texas Southwestern Medical School Library. Denial was the toughest part of the grieving process for us. Reality finally set in when we received the results of the MRI that revealed Emma had enlarged vestibular aqueducts. The idea of our child never hearing music, our voices, birds chirping, television, or movies devastated us.

Our first thought about cochlear implantation was that we would absolutely not put our child through the risks of elective surgery. We accepted Emma as she was and could not fathom the idea of putting her through surgery at such a young age. But after a few months of in-depth research on the benefits of a cochlear implant, we realized that the risks were low when compared to other pediatric surgeries and the rewards were infinite. Further, children tend to recover and bounce back much quicker than adults. Although Emma could detect sound through hearing aids, she could not discern speech well enough to learn to talk intelligibly. At such a young age, it was unlikely that Emma would have learned to talk clearly without the implant.

The decision to go with a cochlear implant was not based so much on our wanting our daughter to hear as it was based on wanting to give Emma a choice; a choice of embracing both hearing and nonhearing worlds. We wanted to give Emma a chance at all options and take maximum advantage of those options. The cochlear implant has maximized her options.

As far as therapy and doctors' appointments go, they have become part of our routine. Life is certainly not boring or uneventful. While we wish Emma could have normal hearing, we must say it has been a journey that has made us all appreciate everything we have.

We were once asked in the days after diagnosis: "If God could put Emma back into the womb and guarantee you she would have all five normal senses but He could not guarantee her personality, would you do it?" Unequivocally the answer would be "No." God could not have made her any more perfect!

—Amy Cook, Emma's mother

Chapter 3

Hearing and How It Is Tested

By Pamela Tunney-Kruger

In this chapter, you will read explanations of the various types of hearing tests that can be done with your child to determine if a hearing problem exists. We will also discuss types of hearing loss, degrees of hearing loss, and, ultimately, the way to come to the best recommendation on how to manage a hearing loss. We begin by explaining who does the testing.

An audiologist is a clinician specially trained in the evaluation, diagnosis, and management of hearing loss. An audiologist has a master's or doctoral level degree, has completed a 1-year externship, and is licensed by the state to assess hearing loss. An audiologist is not a technician but is a fully qualified professional. The audiologist's office, the place where most testing is carried out, is either in a hospital or a clinic. Some of the testing is done in a sound treated room called an audiologic sound suite, whereas other testing is done in a quiet office area.

Hearing Tests

There are many different types of tests that measure how well your child hears. Keep in mind that not all tests are necessarily given to every child. The most important reason to test hearing is to find out the type and degree of hearing loss as efficiently as possible. Each type of hearing test is designed to provide a unique piece of information. The end result of comparing results from different tests is a complete picture of your child's hearing ability. Some tests provide more information than others, and the ability to get that information on a particular test is often affected by how old your child is at the time of testing or how well he is able to participate in some of the testing procedures. Different tests have been designed to be administered with less active participation from your child in the hopes of gathering information earlier in life—even as early as 1 day old.

Behavioral Audiologic Evaluation

Behavioral Observation Audiometry

Behavioral audiologic evaluation can be conducted from infancy to adulthood. Developmentally appropriate procedures are utilized to obtain valid information about hearing sensitivity to tones and speech even from difficult-to-test children. This type of test measures voluntary responses from your child. Because changes in behavior are measured or observed, it is called a behavioral test. For infants 6 months of age and younger, the hearing responses are often described using a procedure called behavioral observation audiometry (BOA). In a BOA exam, the audiologist observes changes in your child's behavior in response to sound. The observed change in behavior could be something as basic as she stops sucking on a bottle or stops crying in response to a sound. It could also include a more sophisticated behavioral change such as turning to look for the source of the sound. A BOA exam is typically appropriate for a very young child or a child who is otherwise unable to participate fully in listening activities. However, BOA responses only provide an informal overview of hearing and/or listening behavior and cannot be used to rule out or confirm hearing loss.

Visual Reinforced Audiometry

A more sophisticated test procedure, called visual reinforcement audiometry (VRA), incorporates a listening activity. This procedure is useful for evaluation of infants from approximately 7 months to

2 years of age. With this procedure, it is possible to determine how loud sounds must be for an infant to hear them.

When a VRA test is done, your child is first taught to listen for a sound and then turn towards the source of the sound. When he does this, he is reinforced or rewarded by seeing an animated or lighted toy appear. This pairing of sound and toy is repeated over and over as different types and loudnesses of sounds are presented. The goal of the test is to find the lowest volume of sound your child will respond to while rewarding him for looking in the direction of the sound by briefly animating a toy.

Conditioned Play Audiometry

Children older than 2 years sometimes become bored very quickly with the animated toys used in VRA. For these children, conditioned play audiometry (CPA) may be used. In this test, your child is taught to respond to the sounds she hears by playing a listening game. For example, she may be asked to drop small toys in a basket each time she hears a sound. As the test proceeds, she continues to play the listening game with sounds at various tones and loudnesses. Usually by the age of 5, children are mature enough to participate in a behavioral audiogram by raising their hand in response to a sound they hear, much like how an adult would respond.

The goal of the behavioral audiogram is to obtain information about the softest level at which a child will respond to tones of various pitches, or frequencies. Typically, the audiologist tries to obtain information for, at a minimum, low frequency (500 Hz) and high frequency (4000 Hz) sounds. The softest level at which the child responds to sounds of various frequencies is plotted on a graph called an audiogram (Figure 3–1).

Sound Field Behavioral Audiogram

When children are very young and participating in a behavioral evaluation, they may not be willing to wear earphones over or in their ears. If that is the case, then their hearing will be tested through a speaker system. Results obtained in this manner comprise a sound field behavioral audiogram. The limitation of sound field testing is that

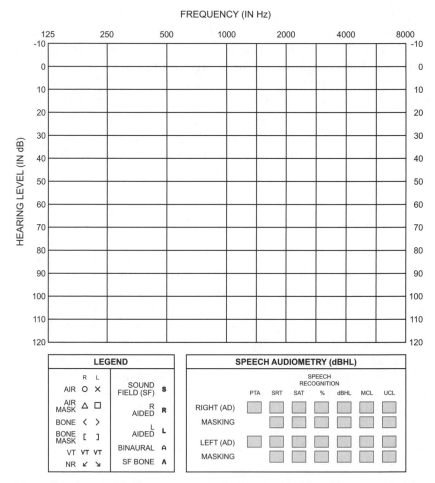

Figure 3–1. A blank audiogram. As each ear is tested with tones or beeps, the responses are recorded on this form with the marks indicated in the key. The pitch of the sound tested (frequency) is on the horizontal and goes from low pitches on the left to high pitches on the right. The loudness (dB) is on the vertical, with the softest sounds at the top of the graph, getting louder as you move down. Speech levels and scores are recorded on the form, too. Courtesy of iStockphoto.com

the audiologist is unable to test each ear separately. If one ear can hear better than the other, a sound field test will not detect the poorer ear's responses. If earphones are used, each ear can be tested individually. If a child is unwilling to wear earphones, as part of the process of ruling out a bilateral (both ear) hearing loss, an audiologist may start with a sound field exam, knowing the limitations, and then making further recommendations as needed.

Terminology

No matter what method is used to test your child's hearing behaviorally, there will be some common terms used to explain the results. Listed here are some of the more common terms used:

- Decibel (dB): A unit of measurement for the loudness of a sound. For example, a 20 dB sound would seem like a whisper level to a person with normal hearing and a 90 dB sound would be very loud to a person with normal hearing.
- Hertz (Hz): A unit of measurement for the pitch or tone of a sound. For example, a 250 Hz tone would have a very deep or bass tone quality, whereas a 4000 Hz tone would have a very sharp or high tone quality.
- Threshold: The softest level at which a person detects a sound. Listed here are the ranges of thresholds for degrees of hearing loss (Figure 3-2).
  - Normal hearing thresholds (0–20 dB)
  - Mild hearing loss (21–40 dB)
  - Moderate hearing loss (41–65 dB)
  - Severe hearing loss (66–95 dB)
  - Profound hearing loss (96+ dB)
- Speech Reception Threshold (SRT): The softest level at which a person can recognize spoken words. As an example, a person with normal hearing should be able to repeat words heard when they are presented at a level of 20 dB or softer.
- Speech Awareness Threshold (SAT): The softest level at which a person is aware that spoken words are present. As an example, a person with a mild hearing loss may have an SAT response as good as 20 dB but not lower than that.
- Word Recognition or Speech Discrimination: A person's ability not only to hear but accurately discriminate one-syllable words at a sufficiently loud level (i.e., conversational speech level). A speech discrimination score of 90 to 100% would be

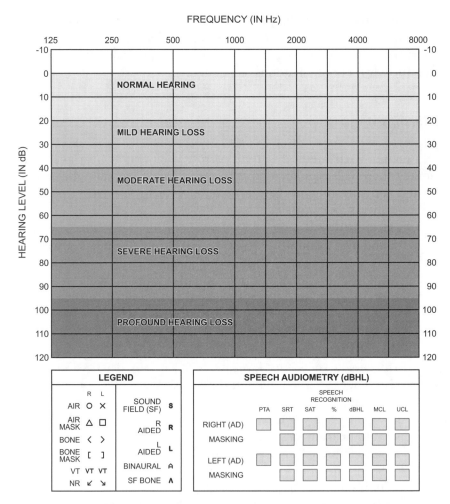

Figure 3–2. Levels of hearing loss. Hearing loss is categorized by five levels of hearing: normal, mild loss, moderate loss, severe loss, and profound loss. Courtesy of iStockphoto.com

good, a score of 80 to 90% would be fair, and below 80% would be poor (Figure 3–3).

▓ Air Conduction: A measurement whereby a test signal is introduced into the ear canal, usually via earphones, and all portions of the ear (outer, middle, and inner ear) participate in hearing the signal.

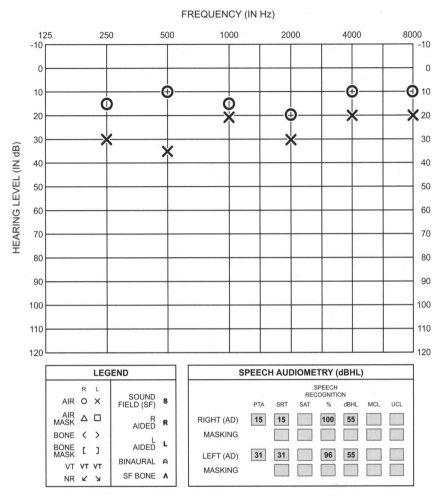

Figure 3–3. Speech scores are recorded on the audiogram in the appropriate boxes. Courtesy of iStockphoto.com

▨ Bone Conduction: A measurement whereby a test signal is presented directly to the cochlea (inner ear) by vibrating the bones of the skull with a small oscillator attached to a headband.

▨ Masking: A signal that is presented to the opposite ear from the one being tested to distract that ear from hearing the test signal. Typically, in cases where one ear may hear markedly better than the other (Figure 3–4), a sound presented to the poorer ear may be loud enough to cross through the skull and be heard by the better ear. A masking signal presented to the better ear will reduce the chance of that ear hearing the test sound.

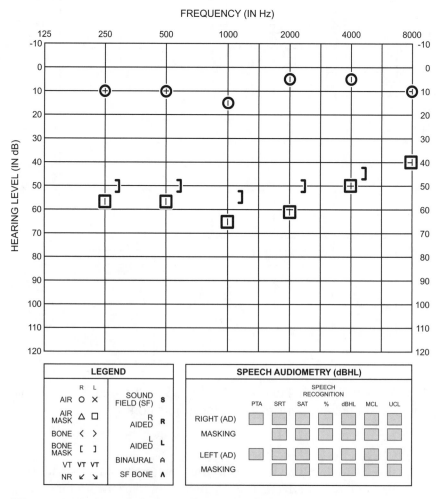

Figure 3–4. A pure tone audiogram showing that the left ear was tested with a masking noise in the right ear. The right ear is masked so it won't hear the tone presented to the left ear. Courtesy of iStockphoto.com

▧ Insert Earphone: A test earphone that has a small foam tip on the end that can be compressed and then placed in the external ear canal (Figure 3-5).

▧ Circumaural Earphone: An earphone that rests fully over the outside of the ear with no portion going into the ear canal (Figure 3-6).

▧ Bone Oscillator: A testing instrument that typically is placed on the mastoid bone behind the pinna (external ear). Sound is transmitted through vibration of the bone. This test allows for

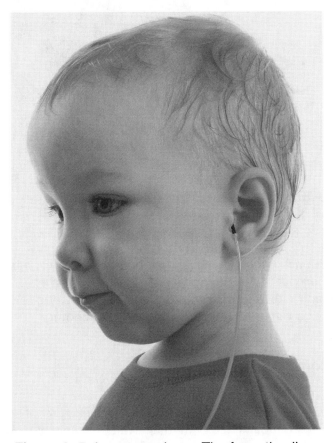

Figure 3–5. Insert earphone. The foam tip allows the earphone to fit snugly in the ear canal. Courtesy of iStockphoto.com

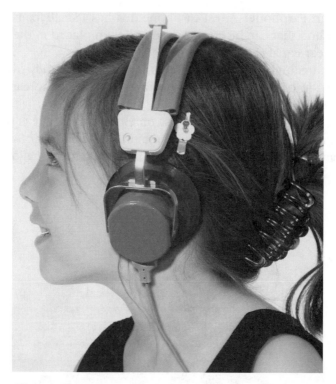

Figure 3–6. Circumaural headphones. Courtesy of iStockphoto.com

additional differential diagnosis of where in the ear a hearing loss may be originating (Figure 3-7).

▪ Sound Field: A term that describes the presentation of a signal through a speaker system within a sound booth.

Tympanometry

Another type of test that is commonly part of the battery of audiologic tests is called tympanometry. Another name for tympanometry is an immittance exam. During this test, the condition of the middle ear is being examined. This test is able to show how well your child's tympanic membrane (eardrum) moves in response to a small amount of

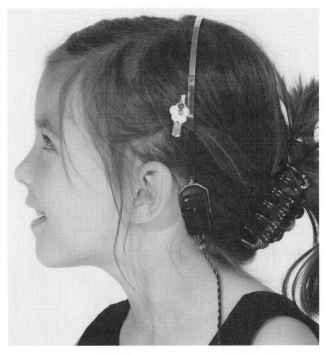

Figure 3–7. Bone conduction headset with the oscillator resting on the mastoid bone. Courtesy of iStockphoto.com

pressure. Your child will probably feel a small change of pressure, similar to what you might feel when you go up several floors in an elevator. The test results produce a graph, called a tympanogram (Figure 3-8), which the audiologist can interpret to reflect how well the eardrum is moving. If your child has had tubes placed in the eardrums, tympanometry can also detect whether a tube is blocked or if it is open and allowing air to pass through.

A second part of the immittance exam is called acoustic reflex testing. During this part of the test, an earplug is placed in one or both ears and a very short but loud sound is presented. Your child does not have to respond in any way. The audiologist is measuring a response from a muscle in the middle ear. The pattern of those responses at different pitches will add to the information collected from your child's other hearing tests.

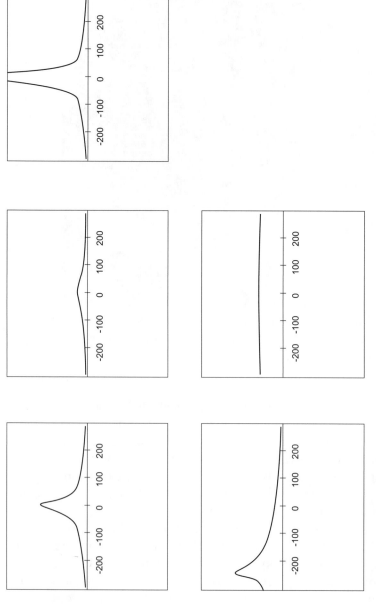

Figure 3–8. Various tympanogram results. Top left is a normal (type A) result. The middle top is a type A$_S$, indicating a stiff eardrum. The top right result is a very flaccid ear drum (type A$_D$). Bottom left is a type C result indicating negative pressure in the middle ear space. The bottom right is a type B or flat result typical of impacted cerumen, eardrum perforation, or middle ear effusion.

Otoacoustic Emissions

Another procedure that is routinely a part of your child's testing is called an otoacoustic emission (OAE) test. There are three types of otoacoustic emission testing: spontaneous, transient, and distortion product. During this exam, a small earplug is positioned in the outer portion of the ear canal. Inside this earplug are a measuring microphone and a small speaker to generate a sound. Sounds enter the outer, middle, and inner ear. In response to this, the ear can generate a measurable response. The recording microphones pick up the small sounds coming back from the inner ear, and a computer averages and processes the responses, displaying the results on the computer screen for interpretation (Figure 3-9).

One of the many advantages to this test is that it usually only takes a few minutes to administer. Your child needs to be in a quiet state, but it is not necessary that she be sleeping. Because each ear is tested individually, we learn more about the function of each ear. An OAE test cannot be used to fully define hearing thresholds, but when used in conjunction with other tests, OAE findings can provide useful information in the overall picture of how your child hears.

Objective Measures of Hearing

Automated Auditory Brainstem Response

In most hospitals today, when children are born, they will have a hearing test completed before they are discharged to go home. Even as young as a few hours old, a newborn's hearing can be tested using a method that does not rely on any subjective response. OAEs can be used for this purpose. Another method often used is a test called an automated auditory brainstem response (AABR). This test is particularly useful in a hospital nursery setting because of its portability and specially designed earphones that fit comfortably over your baby's ears, which allow for a more reliable response to be measured. In most cases, the test can be completed in less than 15 minutes, and results can be reported to you as soon as the testing is complete.

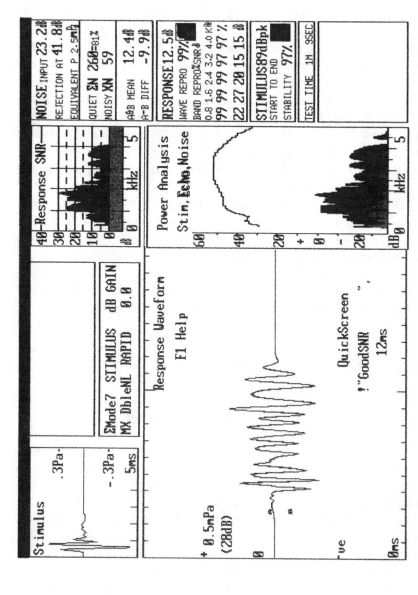

Figure 3–9. Results of the OAE testing displaying the computer averaged responses.

If your baby does not pass the screening criteria, additional testing will be recommended. These tests are important because the first test administered is usually only a screening. Whereas a screening can rule out a hearing loss, it does not test for all possible outcomes. In particular, if your baby fails the screening, there may be a temporary condition causing a hearing loss or there may be a more permanent reason. In order to verify the reason for the failure, additional testing that is more detailed can be completed.

Auditory Brainstem Response

When a newborn does not pass AABR or OAE screening, the result is often confirmed with a diagnostic auditory brainstem response (ABR) evaluation. The ABR is a test of the auditory nervous system. The ABR test can be completed while your child sleeps naturally or is mildly sedated. Electrodes, or sensors, are placed on the child's head (Figure 3–10) to collect the brain's response to sounds. This test is especially useful for the testing of very young or difficult-to-test children. Each ear can be tested individually. Earphones are used to deliver

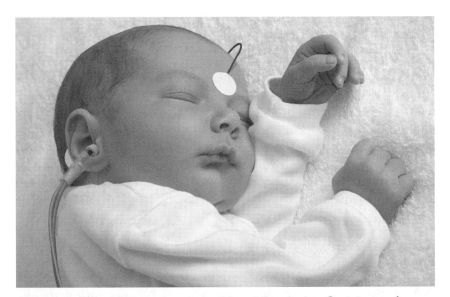

Figure 3–10. ABR test set up with resting baby. Courtesy of iStockphoto.com

sounds at various frequencies and different loudness levels. While the sound is being delivered to the ear, changes in the brain wave patterns (EEG responses) are measured through the sensors and analyzed for a response to the sound. If the responses can be measured at very soft presentation levels, then hearing can be classified as normal. As the loudness of the sounds is adjusted, the degree of hearing loss can be determined. There are two types of sounds that can be used in an ABR test. A click ABR is most sensitive to hearing in the higher frequencies. A tone burst ABR can provide information about hearing at more specific frequencies, most often the low and mid frequency sounds. Combined, these two types of ABR can document hearing abilities across a wide range of frequencies in each ear individually for any age child (Figure 3-11).

It is important to note that neither AABR nor ABR testing can determine how your baby will process or understand what he hears. These tests give information only about the ear's ability to detect a sound. Actual speech understanding, or measurement of how your child processes what is heard, can't be done until he is older and able to participate in more interactive measurements (behavioral audiologic evaluation).

Types of Hearing Loss

In the course of having a child's hearing evaluated, one of the most common questions asked is, "Why can't my child hear normally?" One way to answer that question is to have very specific tests for the many different areas of the ear and the auditory processing centers of the brain. As testing techniques become more sophisticated, they also become more specific to different areas of the inner ear and the regions of the brain that process sound. The basic types of hearing loss are as follows.

Conductive Hearing Loss

For this type of hearing loss, sounds are not transmitted or "conducted" through the ear canal, tympanic membrane, and/or middle ear. This may be due to too much earwax, something else blocking the outer ear, fluid in the middle ear, or a variety of other problems.

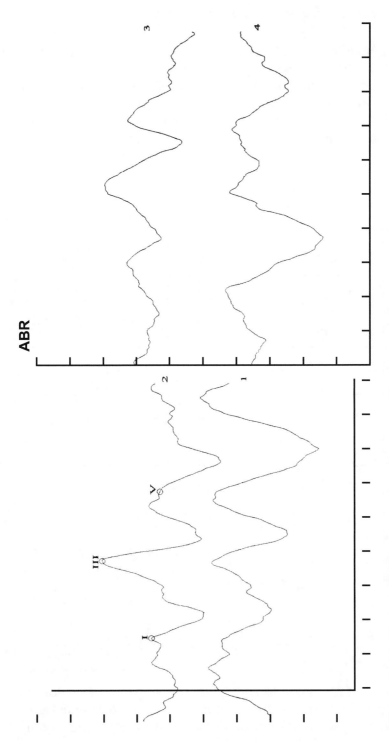

Figure 3–11. Typical ABR tracings showing normal hearing responses.

On the audiogram, the bone conduction responses will be within normal limits, but there will be a hearing loss by air conduction. Conductive hearing loss may be alleviated medically or surgically (placement of pressure equalization tubes). If the conductive hearing loss cannot be resolved medically or surgically, the child may benefit from a hearing aid(s) (Figure 3–12).

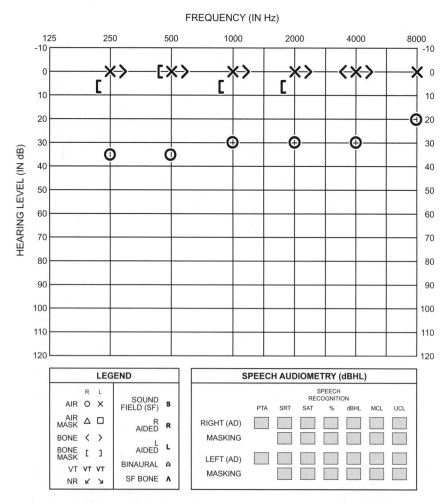

Figure 3–12. Pure tone audiogram showing conductive loss in the right ear. Note that the left ear received a masking noise as indicated by the bracket symbol. Courtesy of iStockphoto.com

Sensorineural Hearing Loss

This hearing loss is due to a problem with the sensory cells in the inner ear (cochlea) or the auditory nerve. This may be caused by heredity, infections, some medications, diseases, and other causes. In many cases, you may never know what caused the hearing loss. Such a hearing loss cannot be resolved with medicine or surgery (unless the child is a candidate for cochlear implantation). If your child has a sensorineural hearing loss, a hearing aid should be considered. On the audiogram, the bone conduction responses and the air conduction responses will both be consistent with hearing loss (Figure 3-13).

Mixed Hearing Loss

Mixed hearing loss, as the name suggests, is a combination of conductive and sensorineural hearing loss. On the audiogram, there is a hearing loss by bone conduction and by air conduction, but the hearing loss by air conduction is worse than that by bone. The conductive component of this hearing loss may be able to be resolved medically, but the sensorineural component may still need to be treated with hearing aids (Figure 3-14).

Auditory Neuropathy

Test techniques utilized by physicians and audiologists can differentiate response regions from different areas within the cochlea itself and through the pathways that carry sound to the brain. Because of the improved specificity of these tests, one diagnosis that can be made (besides the types of peripheral hearing loss described above) is called auditory neuropathy (AN). AN is a hearing disorder caused by poor timing of the auditory nerve. A person with AN may have difficulty understanding speech or learning speech through the normal course of hearing. A child with AN has difficulty because speech does not sound clear on a consistent or regular basis.

Tests that currently best differentiate AN from other causes of impaired hearing function are the ABR evaluation and OAE testing. When done together, the interpretation of the results can lead to more clearly defined understanding of how the ear is behaving.

One of the greatest challenges to making the diagnosis of AN is the variability in test results over time. It is very important to have

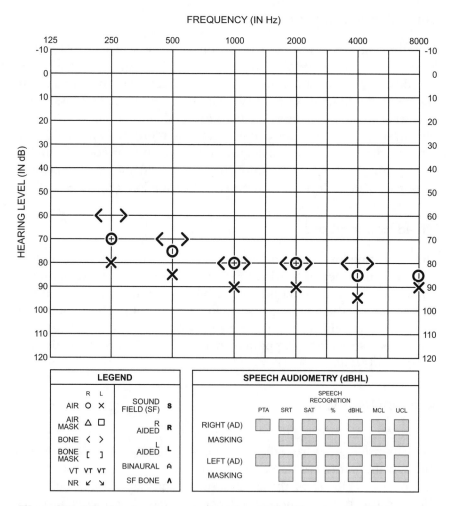

Figure 3–13. A pure tone audiogram indicating a severe sensorineural hearing loss in both ears. Courtesy of iStockphoto.com

your child's hearing monitored very closely by your audiologist so that if changes occur in how the ear is responding, appropriate recommendations regarding intervention can be made.

The management recommendations for AN vary and can include fitting of hearing aids, use of FM systems, cochlear implantation, and sign language and or cued speech. Recommendations may change over time as a result of how stable the condition appears, as well as how well your child responds to the treatment prescribed.

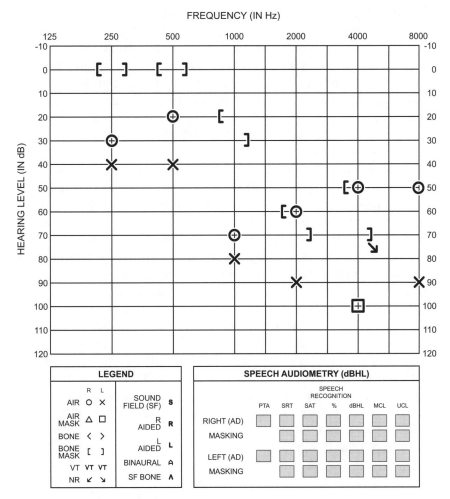

Figure 3–14. A pure tone audiogram showing a mixed loss in both ears. Courtesy of iStockphoto.com

Specialized Testing for Cochlear Implant Recommendation

The choice between implanting one or both ears is often a difficult one. Today, doctors and parents are discussing this option in greater detail. Recent research into binaural hearing through cochlear implants (cochlear implants in both ears) compared to monaural implantation (use of a single implant) has shown improved hearing in noisy environments and improved ability to know the direction of where sound is coming from. In most instances of cochlear implantation, improving speech discrimination and achieving age-appropriate language development milestones are the highest priority. Testing can be done that shows how the pathways of hearing between the inner ear and the brain can improve over time. These changes can be measured in similar ways to how the ABR test is administered. The specific measurement in this case is called the P1 cortical auditory evoked potential. This response can be monitored over time. Studies have shown that after implantation, the response can change from a delayed response to one that is consistent with that of a normal hearing person. Not only does the implant stimulate the ear for hearing, but other neurological changes can occur over time within the ear and auditory pathways.

In conclusion, it is always important to know the reasons why tests are recommended as well as understand the information resulting from those tests. As you work with your doctors, audiologists, and medical caregivers, you will find yourself asking many questions and seeking explanations about how your child hears. Sometimes the answers will be very definitive and other times they may only lead to more questions. Because there are a variety of tests that can be given, they each serve a unique purpose. Keep in mind that not every test is appropriate or necessary for every child. As a parent, however, one can take comfort in knowing that because of the diversity of the tests, your questions can and should be answered. In turn, you can make the important decisions necessary for your child.

Chapter 4

Don't the Insurance People Understand? This Is *My Child*!

By Marjorie K. Maier

Frustration and confusion with your insurance carrier and its processes will be a significant aspect of your journey through your child's cochlear implantation. There are several tools that will help you successfully navigate this aspect of your child's care. We will review the purpose and perspective of the insurance carriers, their role, your role, the physician's role, the role of other health care providers, and the role of office personnel at the physician's office in this cochlear implantation process. Understanding the viewpoint of the insurance company does not mean you will agree with it or like it; however, it will benefit you to recognize that their goals and objectives are not always parallel with your goals. Understanding the roles of the health care providers and office staff will help you and them successfully navigate the insurance maze and achieve the desired end of cochlear implantation for your child.

Understanding the Insurance Carrier

Insurance—The Basics

Most health insurance companies, health plans, health insurers, and carriers are for-profit companies who have a responsibility to their owners and shareholders to remain profitable. The business of insurance is, by nature, one of risk taking. The insurance carrier or health plan takes a risk that the number of relatively healthy people it insures will outnumber the seriously ill people it insures, thereby allowing it to make a profit by paying out less money in health benefits than it takes in as health care premiums. This basic principle is true of health insurance, homeowners insurance, and other common forms of insurance. Most health insurance is purchased by an employer, and eligible employees then choose to enroll themselves and dependents (spouse, children) in the health plan offered by the employer. This is frequently called commercial insurance coverage. Employers buy insurance with various types of coverage, different benefits, and varied levels of care based on what they perceive to be the best value for their employees, and based on what they can afford. Just as you go to the grocery store with a general idea of the types of items you need and what your budget is to cover the cost of these items, employers do the same when buying health insurance for employees. Employers have to choose what to purchase and what fits in their budget. When you are at the grocery store, you may want to purchase the finest steak available, but you may opt for a medium grade of beef or even chicken because those items are more in line with your budget for food. Employers make similar choices when buying health insurance for employees; they may want to buy every type of coverage available but may opt to purchase only those types of coverage they can afford. Unfortunately, the coverage options for hearing devices, cochlear implants (CIs), and other hearing-related equipment and services are often ones that aren't purchased by all employers when they chose what to buy.

Health plans and insurance companies do not have a responsibility to provide every conceivable type of health service or health care for each individual they insure, if that level of coverage or service was not purchased by the employer as part of the health coverage. Similarly, your chicken purchased at the store won't magically turn into fine steak simply because you'd like it to; what you purchased is what you will have to work with in preparing a meal; similarly, what your employer purchased is what you have to work with for insurance for your child. However, health insurance companies and health plans do have a responsibility to provide these services if they are within the scope of the health insurance, and you are your child's best advocate to make this happen. Keep in mind, the insurance carrier has a goal to remain profitable, so any administrative processes that decrease the likelihood that CI monetary benefits will be paid by the insurance carrier actually help it meet its financial goal. You will find many of these administrative processes as you begin seeking insurance coverage for CI services. Some of these processes may seem like obstacles or silly hurdles. Some are actually geared toward gathering and evaluating medical data about your child's health. The processes may help the health plan determine if a service is appropriate and medically necessary and answer a myriad of other questions to determine if the service or item meets its requirements. I am not saying that every health plan process to "meet the requirements" is a needless barrier to care or payment, but each obstacle in the process, each step you have to make, each form that has to be filled out and approved, does decrease the likelihood that you will stay in the race long enough to get the benefits paid for, which is your ultimate goal. This is the point where your role as parent advocate is crucial. Remember, you are the person with the relationship with the insurance company; you or your child is the "covered member" of the health plan. In the simplest of terms, you or your employer bought a service or product from the health plan, so you and your employer are the "customer" of the health plan. Your doctor or audiologist is not in the same customer relationship with your health plan. Physicians and other health care providers choose to participate or "enroll" to be a provider with a health plan. There may be thousands of providers on your health plan's provider list, all who are deemed qualified by your health plan to provide services to covered members of the health plan.

This is similar to your car insurance. If you are in a car accident, there may be a list of approved repair shops through your car insurance. The repair shop seeks payment from the insurance company for services rendered, but you are the actual customer of your car insurance company, not the repair shop. You are a stronger advocate with your car insurance company if there is something about the car repairs that you want to discuss or question, such as how much it will pay, what repairs it'll cover and which it won't, or if it is willing to repaint the whole car or just part of the car after the repair is completed. The repair shop is simply the mechanism for getting the car repairs completed. The repair shop isn't the policy holder or direct customer who has purchased a service through the car insurance company; you are. The same is true for your health insurance plan: you are the customer, not the physician or audiologist or health care provider.

Health Plan—Their Role

Once your physician and audiologist have determined your child is a good candidate for a CI, the first contact with the insurance plan will likely be initiated by your physician's office. The office will contact your insurer to determine eligibility and benefits for these particular services. This determination may be done over the phone or via a fax machine. It should be treated as a preliminary predetermination and not considered the final verdict for your coverage. The health plan or insurance carrier will have a lengthy and specific process with established steps to obtain a full and comprehensive determination of benefits for your child for CIs. The health plan has a responsibility to explain to you what its process is, in what sequence the various steps need to occur, how required information needs to be submitted to it for review, and a time frame for each step in the process. Its role is to explain its approval process and then follow the prescribed process. The rest is up to you and your care team.

After your child is identified as a candidate for a CI, call your employer's benefits office (usually part of human resources) and request a booklet that outlines in detail the coverage limitations of your health insurance. If the benefits office does not have it readily available to give to you, ask it to request it from the health plan on your behalf. The health plan may allow you to access your specific employer benefits on the health plan Web site as well, but ensure that you are reviewing your specific employer's plan benefits. Remember, your employer purchased a few items from the insurance company "grocery store" and you need to look at only what your employer purchased, not what the health plan may have offered for purchase; the information needs to be specific to your benefits through your employer-sponsored health insurance. The health plan does have to supply you with these data about your insurance coverage. Read the booklet or Web page, and focus on information related to hearing services and devices and prosthetics. You may even want to bring a copy to your physician's office to share with the office manager.

Next, call your insurance carrier and ask to speak to the case management department. Ask to speak with a supervisor and request that she explain to you the process for preapproval for a surgical procedure for your child. Obtain names of those you speak to, and document the dates and times of all communication via phone with your insurance plan. It may take more than one phone call to reach a supervisor in case management "in person," but persist until you reach someone who is helpful in explaining the process to you. Request that she fax the information to you outlining the approval process and the steps necessary to request a service or surgical procedure. The steps in the approval process are to be made available to you by your insurance plan; the health plan must provide you with information about the process and it should not be withheld from you because you are a covered member of the health plan. Most health plans have time frames or deadlines associated with the various steps in the approval process; obtain these time deadlines and time requirements, in addition to the steps in the process. It will be important to provide information and respond to the health plan requests within its established time frames. If you don't see it readily available in the information provided by your health plan, also ask about the mailing address to submit medical information, including the name of the medical director and names of reviewers in case management or the predetermination department. Specific names and addresses will be important so mail isn't sent "to whom it may concern" or to a mailing address used for building utilities, such as phone or electric bills, or general business correspondence at the insurance company.

Most health plans will have several supervisors in the case management area; keep calling until you reach one who you find to be friendly and helpful over the phone. Keep returning to the health plan employees who help you and give you information you request. They will be a great resource on this journey, as they will know other helpful people at the health plan in other departments if you need to speak with other people in this process. Think of the case management supervisor as the hub on a wheel who can help you get to spokes on the insurance company wheel when you need them. Above all else, remember you want these people to help you, so be courteous, friendly, and appreciative along the way. Nothing will end your calls faster with the health plan than a rude, angry approach to the employees. Nothing will delay your approval process more than refusing to follow its prescribed steps in the process. When you are overwhelmed and want to scream at them, "This is my *child*; don't you understand?" they will be thinking in their heads, "This is our *process*; don't you understand?" Avoid this stalemate; keep it professional and cordial. At all times, remain respectful of the employees and processes, and do remember to personalize your child to them in an appropriate manner; it won't hurt for them to know your child loves soccer or painting.

Once you are armed with the health plan coverage details and the approval process of your health plan, you are ready to go to work with your health care team including the physician, audiologist, speech-language pathologist, social worker, nurse, and office and billing staff. Refer to Figure 4–1 for more information about the various processes you may encounter as you seek insurance approval for CIs for your child.

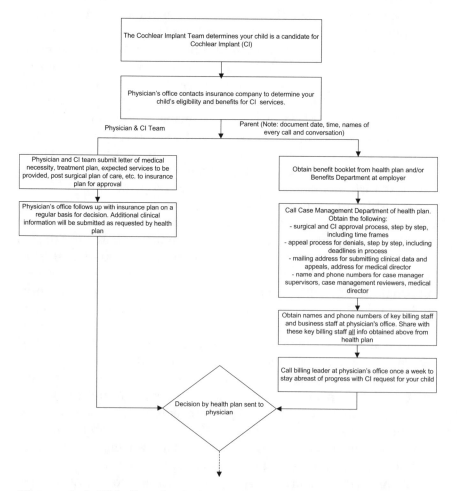

Figure 4–1. This flowchart shows the many steps involved in obtaining insurance coverage for a cochlear implant and all related services. *continues*

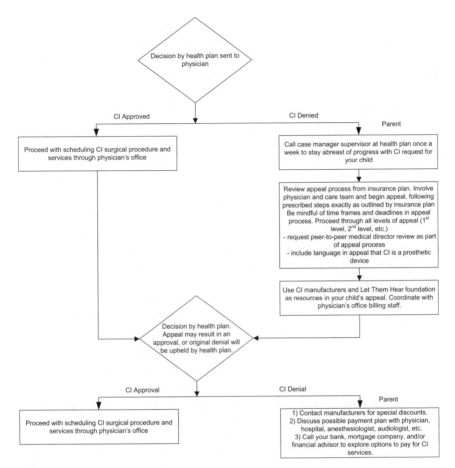

Figure 4–1. *continued*

Medicare and Medicaid

If your child is not covered by a health insurance plan through you or a family member's employer, your child may be covered under the federal Medicare program or the state Medicaid program, both of which are health care plans providing health care benefits to enrolled members or participants on the plan. If you have Medicare or Medicaid coverage, it too will have an approval process to complete prior to approval for cochlear implantation of your child.

The Medicare and Medicaid approval processes may vary slightly from that of commercial insurance coverage discussed above, but many of the basic steps in the process are similar. Both Medicare and Medicaid include CIs as part of the coverage package; they are a "covered benefit" to enrollees, but this does not guarantee approval for each and every patient who requests an implant. The approval and authorization process through Medicare and Medicaid is essential and may follow a similar sequence of medical necessity, preauthorization, or precertification discussed above for commercial insurance plans. You may find fewer physicians, audiologists, and other health care team members participate in the insurance plans provided by Medicare and Medicaid, which may limit the care providers available to you under these plans for CI services. Not all physicians participate in all insurance plans. You pick and choose which activities you and your family will be involved with such as church, sports, school activities, parent groups, and vacations based on how much value those activities have for you and your family. Another factor in your decision is the cost of these various activities and the financial realities of the choices you make. Physicians make similar choices when determining the insurance plans with which to participate. Cost is a factor in their decisions, too. If it costs a doctor $45 to perform a service (cost of staff, supplies, office space, equipment, etc.), and a particular insurance plan is only willing to reimburse $20 for that service, it is doubtful that the physician will participate on that insurance plan. Nonparticipation on a health plan does not mean the doctor is mean or doesn't care about patients; it means she is making a choice based on finances, just as you do when choosing various activities for your family.

If your child is covered by Medicare or Medicaid, their rules and administrative processes will be prescribed by them, and your physician and health care team members will participate in their approval process in similar roles as with commercial payers and insurance carriers.

Money Talk

The harsh reality is that a CI, just like any other device or medical procedure, costs money. It happens to be an expensive technology, and someone has to pay for the device and services. Physicians need to be paid, hospitals need to be paid, audiologists and speech-language pathologists need to be paid, as do the other health care team members involved in your child's care.

Insurance plans have to pay for many health conditions, treatment, care, and devices, and they are stretching their dollars as far as they can while still reaching profits demanded by their owners. Health plans tend to provide more coverage for illness and health issues that are high volume and less coverage for low volume illness and health issues; this is not true in all cases, but is a good general rule of thumb. For example, diabetes is a common, high frequency illness in America, and financial coverage for diabetic care such as physician services, hospital services, and related services is abundant. According to the American Diabetes Association, 20.8 million children and adults in the United States, or 7% of the population, have diabetes (American Diabetes Association, 2008).

Candidacy for CIs is less common than diabetes in America, making it a lower volume health issue for most insurance carriers. According to the National Institute on Deafness and Other Communication Disorders (NIDCD), approximately 59,000 people worldwide have received CIs, and about 250,000 people would be good candidates for the implant (NIDCD, 2008). This does not imply that diabetic care is more important than care for hearing loss through a CI; it is simply more prevalent and more widely covered as an integral part of a health insurance plan.

If the cost to provide services exceeds what insurance plans will pay for the care rendered, there will be a limited number of physicians and health care teams providing the service to patients. In many instances, the insurance reimbursement or payment for CI services falls short of covering the cost or expenses of the service, making it a financial loss to the physician, hospital, or other providers involved in the care. This reality results in limited numbers of care providers offering these services. Remember, this does not mean it's not a valuable or important treatment or care or service; it is simply not one that is attractive from a financial standpoint for insurance plans that pay the bills, or care providers who are paid at a low rates for their services (Blue Cross Blue Shield of Tennessee, 2008). So, you may be saying to yourself, "If the insurance doesn't want to pay for it because it's expensive and low volume, and not all doctors will provide it because it's expensive and reimbursement for care is low, am I doomed?" The answer is no, you are not doomed. Remember, just because something is high dollar, low volume, and limited in nature does not mean it lacks value.

Think for a moment about a fine piece of artwork—expensive, limited in volume or quantity, but valuable in what it adds to the world and the potential it brings for learning and growth. Your child's CI is like this piece of fine art—it is expensive, limited or restricted, but endless in its potential for your child's future. So, in short, it's worth the hassle and frustration of managing the insurance process and seeking coverage for the CI, despite the hurdles along the way.

The Role of Your Physician and Health Care Team

Your Physician's Role

Your physician will likely be providing the bulk of the documentation requested by your health plan to determine coverage for CIs. It is likely that one of the earliest steps in the insurance process will be for the physician to send a letter of medical necessity to your insurance company. This is a letter written by the physician that spells out a number of things in medical terms: the extent and nature of your child's hearing loss; your child's health history and the interventions that have already been tried; an expected plan of treatment; and the expected services to be performed leading up to surgery, the surgery itself, and post-surgical care by the physician and other health care providers such as an audiologist or speech-language pathologist. The physician may choose to send test results, copies of progress notes, or other parts of the medical record to the insurance carrier along with the letter of medical necessity. Your audiologist, speech-language pathologist, social worker, or other health care provider may also provide information to your physician to include in the letter of medical necessity.

You may be asking yourself this question, "If the physician says my child needs this and it will help my child, doesn't that automatically mean it is medically necessary?" The answer is "Not always." Health plans like to make an independent assessment as to whether or not a procedure is a generally accepted medical practice and is effective in reaching desired results.

Your Health Care Team

Your team will also include key individuals from the physician office who perform billing and insurance-related tasks and activities. These people may be called billing coordinators, billing supervisors, office managers or supervisors, or many other job titles assigned to office staff who work to help physicians and health care team members follow the rules of the various insurance plans and get paid by the insurance plans for the care rendered to patients. These individuals in many cases will compile all the clinical and patient care data and submit them to the insurance plan. Any information or names you obtained from your insurance carrier should be shared with these key billing staff members in your physician's office. The billing staff members will likely have contact names as well, which you can ask them to share with you. For this part of the process, the more information and contact names you and your billing team have, the better. You and they will use every means possible to push the request for your child through the approval process at the health plan.

The insurance or billing employees at your physician's office will likely send the request and letter of medical necessity to your insurance plan for processing. Ask your physician or audiologist for the name of the billing person(s) who will be processing your request. There may be one designated person or a group of two or three people who will be involved in submitting information to the insurance company, tracking its progress, making follow-up phone calls, and eventually receiving information back from the insurance carrier about approval or denial of the requested treatment. Obtain the name and phone number of each person at your physician's office who will be part of this submission and decision process. These billing employees are important teammates in the CI process. It may take several weeks for the insurance company to respond to the request from your physician's office. After the information about medical necessity, test results, and so on are submitted, the insurance company may request additional information that the doctor's office will supply. During this time, I encourage you to communicate regularly with the physician's billing staff and with the insurance company directly. Phone calls are a good way to keep abreast of the status of the request. Remember, document the name of who you talk to on the phone, the date and time of your calls, and the items discussed. Because this could be a lengthy process lasting several weeks, it'll be important for you to have a record of the process instead of relying on your memory. This is an emotional and stressful time for you and your family, and your memory may not be clear when you try to recollect multiple phone calls across several weeks. When talking on the phone with the insurance company, be sure to clarify what step in the approval process your case has reached. Because you have already obtained the approval process in writing, you can follow the various steps of your child's case with the insurance company.

The insurance company, after gathering needed data and following their prescribed approval process, will issue a determination or decision back to the doctor's office. The approval or denial may or may not be sent to you, so open communication with the physicians' office is key. If the CI surgical procedure and related treatment are approved, you will move toward scheduling surgery and related services. There will be several care providers involved in your child's care including, but not limited to, the surgeon, audiologist(s), speech-language pathologist, anesthesiologist, social worker, nurses, and others. If the request for approval is denied, you begin the process of denial management. You need to be aware that many insurance companies will approve a single implant but not two. Bilateral implantation (the use of two implants, one for each ear) is a relatively recent development. Audiologists, speech-language pathologists, and implant surgeons are recommending bilateral implants with increasing frequency as the evidence of their superior effectiveness mounts. However, insurance carriers have not caught up. Consequently, it will be more difficult to get approval for a bilateral (two implants) than for just one. Medicare, for example, will not pay for two implants. The situation with Medicaid is always variable and differs from state to state. A number of large insurance companies have recently changed their policies and now pay for bilateral implants, but there are still a significant number of insurers who will not. The Let Them Hear Foundation (see below) has been especially effective in overturning denials for bilateral implants.

Denials Management

It's Your Right and Your Responsibility

Denials for CIs are not uncommon. No one is as vested in your child's health and treatment as you are. Even the caring, dedicated physicians, audiologists, and other care team members do not have the degree of investment in your child that you do, nor do they have the relationship with your insurance carrier that you do, so it's your role and your responsibility as the insured party to passionately pursue an appeal.

This is where you really become your child's advocate, using all means available to obtain approval from your insurance carrier for the CI.

An appeal may involve having the physician request a peer review by a medical director at the insurance company. The medical director is a physician with whom your physician can talk peer to peer about the medical needs of your child. This is often a successful method for turning a denial into an approval. It is necessary at this juncture to follow exactly those prescribed steps authorized by your insurance carrier. Failure to follow the process or failure to provide data in the defined time frames or in the proper format may result in an administrative denial.

The insurance folks in your doctor's office are a great resource to begin the appeal process. The billing staff at your physician's office have processed appeals before and they can guide you through the process. But don't stop there. Utilize all available resources to help appeal the denial, and keep your physician's office informed at each step.

Types of Denials and Methods for Appeal

The type of denial received will help determine your next course of action. A CI can be denied for a couple of reasons: an administrative reason (because it is not a covered benefit) or because it is not medically necessary. An administrative denial may also result from a failure to provide information to the insurance carrier that it requested to help with its decision making, or it results from information being submitted after a prescribed time frame elapsed. Administrative denials can often be appealed and may require you start the request process all over again, from the beginning. The most common reason we see for a denial is that the insurer claims that cochlear implantation is not a covered benefit. Frequently, this decision can be appealed by describing the CI as an implantable prosthetic device. Medicare covers CIs under this exact definition. The Social Security Act, Section 1861 (s) (8) defines prosthetic devices as "devices (other than dental) that replace all or part of an internal body organ." CIs are classified under this act as a prosthetic device, along with, but not limited to, cardiac pacemakers. Just because Medicare considers it a covered benefit does not guarantee that your particular insurance carrier will cover the surgery and device, but appealing the denial on the basis that it meets the definition of a prosthetic is a good starting point for your appeal. Your physician can help write the language necessary to support this appeal with your insurance plan.

A denial due to lack of medical necessity means the insurance company does not feel the surgery or device is necessary, reasonable, or in keeping with generally accepted practices or meets specific criteria of your health plan. Contact the case management department at your insurance carrier (remember, you have a list of names and phone numbers of helpful people in that department) and ask that you be sent its specific definition of *medically necessary*. This will help guide your care team and particularly your physician as a letter is written to appeal the decision that the CI is not medically necessary. The letter of appeal can directly address the specific elements of medical necessity as defined by your particular insurance plan. The more closely your appeal matches their policies and processes, the more effective your appeal will be.

Appealing adverse decisions issued by the insurance plan can be a lengthy process. It often involves submitting paper documentation in addition to phone calls between your physician and a physician representative at the health plan. It may take several additional weeks to appeal a denial, which prolongs an already drawn-out process. Help in appealing an adverse decision is provided to patients and parents by all three CI manufacturers and by the Let Them Hear Foundation. The Let Them Hear Foundation is an independent, legal service that has been very successful in getting denials for both unilateral and bilateral implants overturned. Appealing a denial, however, is your right as a covered member of the health plan and a responsibility if indeed you and your health care team believe cochlear implantation to be appropriate for your child.

Additional Resources

There are three manufacturers of CI devices; in alphabetical order they are Advanced Bionics, Cochlear Corporation, and Med-El. Your physician has probably talked to you about all three manufacturers and the various aspects and features of each device. It is likely at this point that you, in partnership with your care providers, have selected a particular device and manufacturer for your child. Each manufacturer has an insurance office or reimbursement department that focuses on helping patients navigate the denial process to obtain approval from an insurance carrier for a CI. You may contact them as follows:

Advanced Bionics Reimbursement Service Department, toll-free phone (877) 779-0229; TTY (800) 678-3575; E-mail: insurance@advancedbionics.com

Cochlear Corporation Reimbursement Department, toll-free phone (800) 633-4667; E-mail: reimbursement@cochlear.com

Med-El Reimbursement Department, toll-free phone (888) 633-3524; V/TDD (888) 633-3524; E-mail: reimbursement@medelus.com

These resources at the manufacturers are a great supplement to the team of billing and insurance staff members at your physician's office. Use both resources, but be sure to coordinate efforts so there is no duplication of effort or conflicting data submitted by either party on behalf of your child.

Let Them Hear Foundation

Another resource for denial management is an organization called Let Them Hear Foundation. Their Web site is http://advocacy.letthem hear.org/ This organization provides a number of services, including assistance with appealing a denial from your insurance carrier. Contact it directly to begin the application process for its assistance. Again, coordinate with your physician's office.

Your physician's office and these various community resource and manufacturer groups must be working cooperatively on your child's behalf in order to effectively turn a denial into an approved surgical procedure at your insurance carrier. Your physician and health care provider team are the people who can provide medical data to support your appeal with the insurance plan. These medical data partnered with the resources of community groups may speed the process of appealing a denial. Most health plans have several levels of appeal, such as first level, second level, and final level of appeal. Do continue to appeal your case until you have fully exhausted all levels of appeal within your health plan. Don't stop if your appeal is not successful at the first level. Persevere, follow the exact process outlined by the health plan, involve the medical care team, and access available resources.

If after the full appeal process you remain unable to have the CI paid for by your health plan, appeal to the various manufacturers for any special programs they may offer for underinsured patients. Other options include arranging a payment plan with the hospital, doctor's office, and other providers involved with the CI so you may pay for the device and services over time. Consult your local bank, mortgage company, or financial advisor to explore other options to finance CI services not covered by your insurance plan.

References

American Diabetes Association. (2008, May 14). *About diabetes.* Retrieved May 14, 2008, from http://www.diabetes.org/about-diabetes.jsp

National Institute on Deafness and Other Communication Disorders. (2008, April 8). Hearing statistics. Retrieved May 14, 2008, from http://www.nidcd.nih.gov/health/statistics/hearing.asp

Blue Cross Blue Shield of Tennessee, Inc. (2008, January 4). Medical Policy Manual (public document). Retrieved May 14, 2008, from http://www.bcbst.com/providers/manuals

Scooter's Story

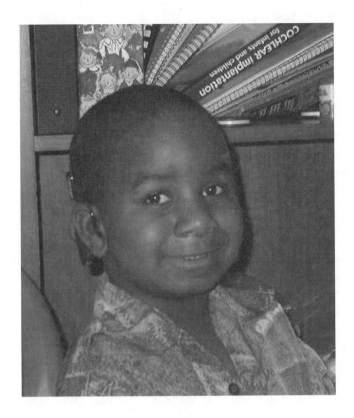

Scooter (his nickname) was a lively 1½-year-old, learning how to speak and spending lots of time with his grandmother and grandfather. One particular weekend, on Friday, his grandmother noticed Scooter wasn't acting like himself. She watched him for a while as he sat in front of the TV. When his grandfather came in the room and had to touch him on the shoulder to get his attention, the look on Scooter's face told her what she feared: Scooter couldn't hear.

Trying to convince Scooter's mom wasn't easy at first. She said, "Oh, he's just not paying attention to you. He can hear."

When Scooter's mom came to pick him up that afternoon she said, "Just wait until he hears my car keys rattle. He'll jump up and be ready to go home." This is what he had always done before.

But Scooter didn't jump up. And then mom knew, too, that something was wrong. On Saturday, the whole family watched

Scooter, trying to pick up telltale signs of hearing behavior. None were seen. On Sunday, his grandmother took him to the emergency room. Surely they'd be able to tell them what was wrong.

At the emergency room they couldn't find anything wrong and claimed he must be having a reaction from an ear infection. Grandmother was too smart for that. She knew how children behaved when their ears hurt. Scooter showed no such behavior.

On Monday, the family called Children's Medical Center's ear, nose, and throat clinic to get an appointment. It was going to be over a month before they could see him. Grandmother insisted that he be seen sooner than that. "He's in trouble! He can't hear!" The woman on the phone heard the urgency in her voice and asked grandmother, "How soon can you bring him in?"

"Right now!"

"His hearing is zero," the audiologist said. Sure enough, Scooter was deaf. One of grandmother's first thoughts was how was this little man going to make it on his own?

Scooter received a cochlear implant about a year later when he was 2½. The Early Childhood Intervention counselor who came to the house was a godsend, according to the grandmother. "She made recommendations about treatment, school placement, and anything else we needed. She was the one who suggested cochlear implantation and got us to our cochlear implant center. She was there for the surgery and for Scooter's hookup. She went through everything with us."

"Very soon we knew the cochlear implant was helping. You could tell when Scooter could hear because he gets a smile on his face. He had only one implant at first so all sound was coming through just one side. He learned quickly that sound could be coming from anywhere, not just on the side where he heard it. He would rapidly turn his head from left to right trying to figure out where the sound was coming from. It was easy to tell when he was listening," says grandmother.

By the time Scooter was 4 he stopped wearing the body-worn processor and started wearing one behind the ear, like the big kids. Much to the consternation of his family, Scooter learned how to turn his CI off and on and to change batteries, too. They had to hide the batteries because he could tell when they were just beginning to go bad and he would change them too soon. "You need to get all you can out of them because they aren't cheap!" When he didn't want to mind his grandmother he'd turn his CI off.

"I told you not to do that! Why did you turn it off?"

"I didn't want to hear you today." He was a regular child!

Scooter received a second implant when he was 6 years old. There were some initial adjustment problems and he didn't get to wear both at the same time for a while. He was anxious and ready for both, and when he finally got to wear them at the same time he seemed to have no difficulty.

"Scooter is doing fine in school. The family is at peace with his life right now because they know he can make it on his own. God has blessed him and us. The cochlear implant has changed everything!"

—As told by Mama, Scooter's grandmother

Chapter 5

Which Cochlear Implant Device Is Right for Your Child?

By Phillip L. Wilson and Holly S. Whalen

Choosing a cochlear implant (CI) device for your child requires a thorough analysis of the products available and their features. It is also advisable to think about your child's personality and habits in order to match the features of the various implants with the unique needs of your child and family. The decision to choose a particular device involves many considerations, including medical considerations, ease of use, wearing options for infants and toddlers, visual appeal, device warranty considerations, and the cost of replacing nonwarranty parts. Many parents would say that none of these factors is as important as choosing the device that gives your child the "best" chance to learn to listen and recognize speech at near normal listening levels. At this time, there is not a clear choice among implant systems with regard to speech recognition.

Manufacturers of implants are well aware of their competition (other implant manufacturers), and when one company introduces a new feature, that feature is often added to the design of other competing manufacturers. The result is that, over time, each of the manufacturers has products and features that are more or less comparable to all the other products. Still, there are differences in the way that these features may be accessed. It would be wise for you to give the various products thoughtful consideration with respect to the needs of your child and your family.

Hearing, Hearing Loss, and Implants

Before you decide which implant device to choose for your child, it is important to understand how a CI works. In the process of explaining how implants work, we will begin with a discussion of the inner ear (cochlea) and how it processes the sounds we hear. If you know how the normal cochlea works and which parts of the cochlea are not working when there is a permanent hearing loss, then the way a CI works becomes clearer.

Sounds in our environment are vibrations of air molecules. These vibrations are transmitted to the cochlea through a mechanical process in the middle ear. Sound waves (moving molecules) strike the eardrum (tympanic membrane) and are transmitted through the middle ear space by three small bones. These small bones, the malleus, incus, and stapes, are suspended in air in the middle ear by small muscles and ligaments. The last bone in the series, the stapes, fits into the cochlea in an area known as the oval window. When sound causes these bones to vibrate, the characteristics of the sound are carried through the middle ear and onwards to the inner ear (Figure 5-1).

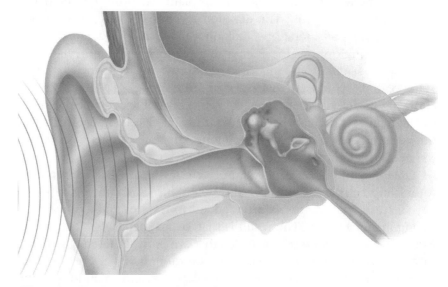

Figure 5–1. Anatomy of the ear. Courtesy of Cochlear Corporation.

The sensory cells of the hearing system are located in the cochlea on a long membrane known as the basilar membrane. The cochlea coils upward from its base to the apex, and the basilar membrane coils with it, suspended in fluid in the cochlea. The vibration of the stapes in the oval window causes the fluid in the cochlea to move. The basilar membrane is flexible, and it moves when the fluid in the cochlea moves. This movement from the base of the cochlea to its apex is called the "traveling wave." The flexibility of the basilar membrane is greater at some locations in the cochlea than it is at other locations. The basilar membrane is stiffer at the base of the cochlea, near the stapes, than it is at the apex of the cochlea. The stiffness of the basilar membrane is one of the mechanisms that enables the sensory part of the ear to distinguish among the complex parts of sound; most importantly, speech.

The basilar membrane supports thousands of sensory cells known as hair cells. There are two types of hair cells: outer hair cells and inner hair cells. Each outer hair cell is connected to a nerve on one end, and the hairs (stereocilia) are embedded in another membrane (tectorial membrane) at the top of the cell. When the basilar membrane moves as a result of the fluid movement caused when the stapes passes the mechanical energy of sound from the middle ear to the cochlea, the stereocilia move, causing a chemical reaction in the hair cell. This chemical reaction causes an electrical event, which then causes the attached nerve to "fire." The firing of the nerve is passed on from the outer hair cell to the inner hair cell.

The stereocilia of the inner hair cells project into the fluid of the inner ear, and if the fluid movement is strong enough the inner hair cells also create a response to the attached nerve cells. The inner hair cells are activated when the fluid movement causes their stereocilia to move enough to cause a chemical reaction to occur in the cell body. Inner hair cells can create their own nerve response, but they also pass on the electrical response of the outer hair cells. The only connection of these sensory cells to the auditory nerve is through the inner hair cells.

In a normal system where all sensory cells are present and functional, the pitch (frequency) of complex sound (like speech) is coded by the variable flexibility of the basilar membrane and by the strength of the traveling wave causing certain hair cells to respond (depending on the frequency of the sounds). High frequency (treble) sounds are specific to the hair cells close to the base of the cochlea. Low frequency (bass) sounds are specific to the hair cells close to the apex. Nerve fibers attached to the hair cells carry specific frequency information. These fibers combine to form the auditory nerve (also known as cranial nerve VIII), and the combined nerve fibers from the cochlea are arranged "tonotopically," or by frequency.

The frequency arrangement of the cochlea and the auditory nerve is very important because it allows individuals to recognize complex speech. Speech sounds are composed of many frequencies from low frequency to high frequency. Vowel sounds in speech are mostly low to mid-frequency. Consonant sounds are mostly mid-frequency to high frequency. In order to recognize words spoken in a sentence, an individual must be able to get enough information from speech to hear all of the critical elements. For example, to recognize the word *cake*, one must hear the high frequency consonants /k/, as well as the vowel /a/. One must also hear the high frequency consonants clearly enough to distinguish the consonants from other similar consonant sounds such as /t/ or /s/, which could make the word seem to be *take* or *case*.

Permanent hearing loss generally results from nonfunctional sensory cells. Whatever the cause, the result is that hair cells do not work as expected. The hair cells themselves may not even be present or they may have been damaged by disease, noise, or ototoxic medication. In general, individuals who have lost functional use of their outer hair cells have a mild to moderate hearing loss. Individuals who have lost both outer and inner hair cells have a severe to profound loss. Individuals who have lost hair cells at the base of the cochlea have high frequency hearing loss. Individuals who have lost hair cells along the entire length of the cochlea have hearing loss at all frequencies.

When significant numbers of functional hair cells exist in the cochlea, a hearing aid may provide adequate stimulation so that the individual can function adequately. In this process, sound is amplified by the hearing aid. Functional hair cells create nerve impulses that signal to the brain that sounds of certain frequency have occurred. In this situation, the hearing aid has increased the intensity of the sound enough to generate a response by the cochlea that the individual can hear and understand.

When populations of hair cells are very low or nonexistent, no level of amplified sound can cause a nervous system response. No matter how loud the signal, if there are no hair cells or limited numbers of hair cells present in the cochlea, the auditory nerve is not stimulated and the individual cannot hear or recognize speech. Individuals who cannot hear or recognize speech with hearing aids may be candidates for CIs. When children are very young and have permanent hearing loss, it is sometimes very difficult to determine whether it would be better to use a hearing aid or a CI. In general, the more severe the loss, the more likely a CI is to be the best treatment. Because implant technology has improved so much in recent years, the criteria for implant candidacy have expanded to include children with less severe hearing loss.

Implant Components

A CI system consists of an internal component and external components (Figure 5–2, Figure 5–3, and Figure 5–4). The internal component includes the receiver-stimulator and the electrode array and is surgically implanted. The receiver-stimulator will be placed in the bone somewhere behind your child's ear, depending on your child's anatomy and the surgeon's technique. It contains a magnet to help keep the external part of the implant system in place. After surgery, in the area where the receiver-stimulator is placed, you may feel a slight bump on your child's head. This will actually be the receiver-stimulator. It is important that you really explore how this feels, so that if the feeling ever changes you will be able to alert your implant center. The electrode array extends from the receiver-stimulator and is implanted into your child's cochlea by the surgeon. It contains multiple channels that, when placed in the cochlea, are responsible for stimulating the acoustic nerve.

The coil or headpiece is an external component that holds a second magnet. It transmits information across the scalp to the receiver-stimulator. It is important to always watch the magnet strength on the coil or headpiece. This can be a balancing act. You want it to be tight enough to keep it on your child's head when your child is walking or playing, but not so tight that it is pulling on the internal component. (If you notice any redness or swelling you should contact your implant center immediately. Not doing so could cause major damage to the flap of skin covering the internal device.) The coil or headpiece receives

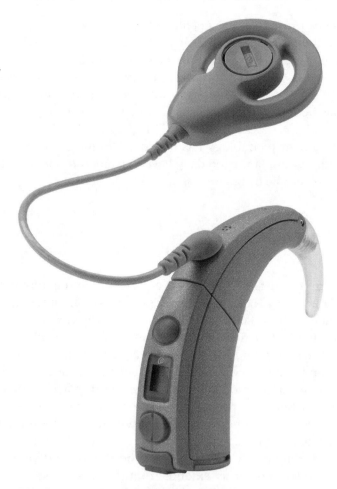

Figure 5–2. Speech processor and headpiece.
Courtesy of Cochlear Corporation.

information from the speech processor. The speech processor is responsible for coding sound in such a way as to make speech recognizable and to allow for identification of environmental sounds.

Depending on the system you choose, the processor will either be located on your child's ear or pinned onto the shoulder or perhaps in a harness. The microphone is usually located on the speech processor. It is important to remember that sound enters the device at the microphone. If you choose to have your child wear the processor

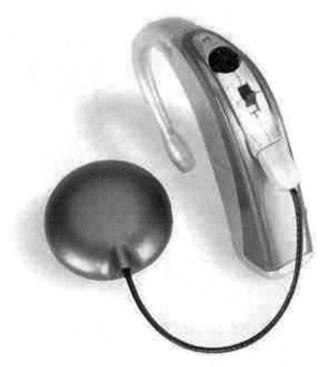

Figure 5–3. Speech processor and headpiece.
Courtesy of Advanced Bionics Corporation.

pinned to the shoulder, then it is important to make sure the microphones are not covered by clothing or other items. A covered microphone will reduce the sound level and speech quality that your child receives from the implant.

The speech processor is powered by batteries. The battery portion of the implant varies between manufacturers. The batteries are either rechargeable or disposable. The disposable batteries are high power 675 batteries, similar to those used in hearing aids. These can be purchased from several different vendors including your child's CI manufacturer. The batteries are a higher power than those generally sold for hearing aids. Importantly, note that a regular hearing aid battery tester should not be used with these batteries. A regular tester might indicate that a battery is good; however, there may not be enough power left to run a speech processor. The rechargeable batteries are designed differently by different companies and cannot be

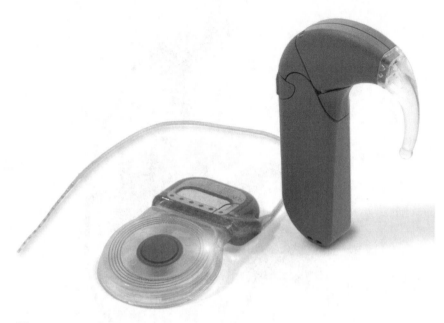

Figure 5–4. Speech processor with receiver-stimulator and electrode array. Courtesy of Med-El Corporation.

interchanged between manufacturer devices. The length of time they last will vary. Rechargeable batteries are available for all three implant manufacturers available in the United States but not necessarily for every battery pack within a manufacturer's line. Batteries may last longer when your child is initially implanted, but as the programming on the speech processor changes, the batteries may give less time between each charge. If the length of time your batteries last changes significantly, it is important to contact your child's CI center. Shortened battery life might indicate that the speech processor needs to be replaced.

How Does an Implant Work?

Sound in the environment is picked up by the implant system microphone. It is then evaluated by the speech processor and coded in a specific way. The coded signal is sent to the coil/headpiece through a cable. The coil is held in place on the head by a magnet that is attracted to the magnet in the receiver-stimulator, just below the skin. The coil sends the coded signal to the receiver-stimulator by FM radio frequency transmission. The coded signal then is processed by the receiver-stimulator and is sent along the electrode array to the cochlea. The receiver-stimulator has divided the coded signal in such a way that the different parts of the signal are sent to the appropriate place in the cochlea. Remember, in the normal hearing ear the hair cells, when adequately stimulated, create an electrical event that causes the nerve to fire. In a CI, the system battery supplies power to the electrode array, which stimulates auditory nerve fibers because of the nearness of the electrode array to the nerve. The electrical signal is sent through the nervous system to the brainstem and on to the hearing centers in the temporal lobe of the brain.

For your child to receive stimulation from the speech processor, all of the different parts must be in place and functioning properly. During appointments your audiologist will make sure all parts of the implant system are in good working order and that cables and connections are in good condition. Based upon observation, testing, and your input as a parent, the audiologist will determine the best way to program your child's speech processor. This is an ongoing process. It is especially important in the beginning to frequently troubleshoot the equipment to ensure that your child is receiving a consistent signal. Changes in programming will be more common in the early part of the process which will stabilize until only minor changes may be needed at subsequent follow-up appointments.

Speech Processing Strategies

Devices and techniques for electrical stimulation of the auditory nerve have been under development for over half a century. Initial negative results have given way to the successful development of processors, providing children and adults with signals that make possible normal language learning and speech recognition ability. A key component in the progress has been improvement in speech processors and speech processing strategies.

The purpose of the speech processor is to produce an electrical copy of speech that can be delivered to the electrode array in the cochlea in such a way that the essential elements of speech are captured by your child's auditory nerve. The electrical stimulation of the auditory nerve by the implant system bypasses the missing hair cells. Implant technology has also taken into account the frequency arrangement of the cochlea by delivering the electrical stimulation to the auditory nerve fibers at the correct location to make speech as clear as possible to the child. If the speech processing strategy is effective and all of the implant components are functioning properly, then your child will have access to the "raw materials" of speech that can aid in language learning, speech recognition, and environmental awareness.

A description of the technical aspects of the various speech coding strategies in current use is beyond the scope of this chapter. As implant manufacturers are constantly attempting to upgrade and improve their strategies, any description would also be quickly out of date. However, a basic goal of speech processing strategies is to transfer the frequency, intensity, and rate of speech to the cochlea, using the frequency characteristics of the cochlea for stimulation of the appropriate auditory nerve fibers. Speech coding strategies are developed considering the important aspects of speech. These aspects include the fact that speech is rapid and complex, that speech sounds do not occur in isolation but overlap with each other, that vowel sounds are composed of simultaneous bands of energy at different frequencies, that consonant sounds have different characteristics based upon the way they are made in the mouth, that many consonants include the use of voice as a distinguishing characteristic, and that nasal elements of speech affect listener perception.

In addition to these factors, which must be considered in coding, speakers can change the meaning of their speech by changing the tone of their voice, by emphasizing certain words, and by changing the rate and pattern of their speech. Because the number of channels and electrodes cannot match the quantity of sensory cells in the normal cochlea, it is impossible to deliver this degree of complexity with a CI. A speech processor cannot simply reproduce speech. For that reason, coding strategies must seek to reduce speech to its essential elements and improve the transmission quality, so that the human nervous system can adapt and use the information for speech recognition. Most strategies currently in use take "real time" samples of speech and convert them into patterns that can successfully be processed in the cochlea. These strategies do not attempt to reproduce every aspect of the speech signal because the hearing loss has reduced the physical capabilities of the ear's processing system.

Each manufacturer of implant systems has a default speech coding strategy that it has implemented to best work with the number of electrodes for its particular device. These strategies are approved by the U. S. Food and Drug Administration for use with children. Although changes may be made to other parameters of the MAP or program, switching coding strategies is done infrequently and on a case-by-case basis.

Continued improvement in speech processing strategies is a goal of all the implant manufacturers, as well as many independent researchers. This research may focus on ways to make use of the remaining physical capabilities of the impaired cochlea by providing more detailed information about frequency and speech structure in ways that can be used by children and adults with CIs.

Implant Features

The three CI companies are Advanced Bionics Corporation, Cochlear Corporation, and Med-El Corporation. They each have different philosophies about electrode arrays, speech coding strategies, and how their speech processors work. When deciding which implant to choose, it is important to first check with your surgeon to see if there are any surgical considerations that would favor one device over another. If the surgeon does not have a surgical preference, then you can choose from the devices available at your center. Not all centers use all three manufacturers.

Table 5-1 compares the three implant manufacturers providing devices in the United States. The various features are described in the text. This table is accurate as of May 2008.

All three manufacturers offer multichannel systems. All manufacturers have both ear level (BTE) and body-worn speech processors. Parents often would like to be told which implant system is best; however, there is no clear answer to this question. There are no studies comparing the most recent devices. All manufacturers have ranges of success with their implants, with some low performers and some "star" performers.

Table 5–1. Comparison of Current Implant Systems

	Cochlear Freedom BTE	Cochlear Freedom Bodyworn	Advanced Bionics Platinum Sound Processor	Advanced Bionics Harmony	Med-El Opus 1	Med-El Opus 2
Internal Component	Nucleus Freedom	Nucleus Freedom	HiRes 90K	HiRes 90K	Pulsar, Sonata	Pulsar, Sonata
Style Options	BTE battery pack, baby worn	Body worn battery pack	Body worn	BTE	5 different wearing options	5 different wearing options
Battery Type	Cochlear rechargeable and disposable batteries	2 AAA (rechargeable or disposable can be used)	Advanced Bionics rechargeable or AA battery pack	Advanced Bionics rechargeable battery	Disposable batteries	Med-El rechargeable and disposable batteries
Programming Options	ACE, SPEAK, CIS, Smart Sound	ACE, SPEAK, CIS, Smart Sound	SAS, CIS, MPS, HiRes-P/S, Fidelity 120	HiRes-P/S, Fidelity 120	CIS, Fine Structure Processing	CIS, Fine Structure Processing
Number of Programs	4	4	3	3	3	3

	Cochlear Freedom BTE	Cochlear Freedom Bodyworn	Advanced Bionics Platinum Sound Processor	Advanced Bionics Harmony	Med-EI Opus 1	Med-EI Opus 2
Controls	Programs, sensitivity, volume, telecoil, ear indicator, lock enabled	Programs, sensitivity, volume, telecoil, ear indicator, lock enabled	Program, volume, sensitivity	Program, volume, or sensitivity knob	Program, sensitivity, volume switch (X, Y, Z)	Programs, volume, and sensitivity are changed using a remote control
Color Choices	Beige, brown, silver, black, pink, and blue	Beige, brown, silver, black, pink, and blue	Silver	Silver, dark sienna, and beige metallic	Anthrocite, Nortic Gray, Sienna Brown, Pacific Blue, Bordeaux Red	Anthrocite, Nortic Gray, Sienna Brown, Pacific Blue, Bordeaux Red
Open MRI	MRI testing to 1.5 tesla with the magnet removed	MRI testing to 1.5 tesla with the magnet removed	MRI testing to 1.5 tesla with the magnet removed	MRI testing to 1.5 tesla with the magnet removed	0.2 tesla with no removal	0.2 tesla with no removal
Alerts	Alerts you to dead batteries, low batteries, coil error, sound/ stimulation error, and corrupt map	Alerts you to dead batteries, low batteries, coil error, sound/ stimulation error, and corrupt map	Alerts you to communication error, low or dead batteries, successful sound transmission, and battery life	Alerts you to communication error, low or dead batteries, successful sound transmission, and battery life	Alerts you to low batteries, processor error, program error	Alerts you to low batteries, processor error, program error

There are a few things to consider when choosing an implant system. One of the most important things to think about is how your child will wear the device. The two main options are a behind-the-ear (BTE) and a body-worn option.

The BTE is worn completely behind the ear, pinned to clothing at shoulder level, or worn with the microphone portion on the ear and the battery pack pinned at shoulder level. When wearing the processor completely behind the ear, "huggies" (plastic rings used to secure the processor to the ear) or earmolds can be used to keep the processor from falling off. You will need to decide if your child's ears are strong enough to hold the weight of the speech processor. If not, you will need to consider pinning the speech processor to the shoulder or you may need to consider a body-worn device. When children are very small, it can be difficult for their ears to sustain the weight of the equipment. As children grow, their ears become larger and firmer, making it easier to keep the equipment in place (Figure 5-5).

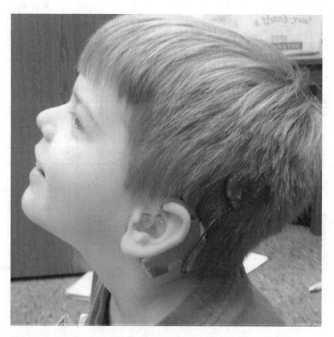

Figure 5–5. Speech processor and headpiece on young boy.

Although pinning the processor to the shoulder and using a longer cable is an option, it is not optimal. When wearing the processor on the shoulder you should be very cautious that the microphone is not covered by a sweater or jacket. This can attenuate or muffle the sound your child is receiving. Also, to face the signal, your child would have to turn his entire body, not just the head.

The microphone on the ear and the battery pack on the shoulder is an option that can often be used in a transition period for children, when they are not quite ready or able to wear the device completely behind their ear. This gives them sound at ear level but takes some of the weight off of their ear. Most implant centers have demo devices that you can try on your child to get a feel for what they will be like. Make sure you try the devices on the ear with the batteries in to get an idea of the weight of the device. Also, make sure to find out if your center offers a one- or two-processor system when making your decision.

The body-worn device has a boxlike speech processor that can be worn on a harness or a belt. Some parents even have undershirts specially made to hold the equipment. Advanced Bionics is currently the only company that offers a strictly body-worn processor.

Another consideration when choosing an implant system is how actively your child will be involved in the day-to-day care and maintenance of his equipment. With multiple wearing options, many different, very small pieces may be a part of your child's implant system. It can be very difficult for children to manipulate small pieces. If your child is old enough to help when picking a system, watch your child manipulate the pieces. Make sure he is able to do tasks like changing the batteries or turning the equipment on and off.

It is also important to consider what parts of your child's speech processor are covered under the warranty. Coils/headpieces, battery packs, and the part of the processing unit with the microphone are generally covered. Cords and batteries are usually not, and if they are they have a limited warranty. If a cord is attached to the coil/headpiece, it is generally covered under the warranty. It is important to consider this because replacement parts can be costly, and if they are covered by your insurance, receiving them can take time. You should also look into any additional warranties that the manufacturer may offer and make sure you renew these policies before expiration. No matter how careful you are, equipment is going to break from time to time. You don't want your child to miss out on being a kid because you are too afraid the equipment might break.

Other Considerations

FM Equipment

Many school programs use FM equipment to improve your child's performance in background noise. An FM system requires the teacher to wear a microphone and transmitter that sends information to a receiver that is worn on the CI. All current speech processors available in the United States are compatible with standard FM equipment. Additional components may be needed to couple the FM system with the speech processor. Speak with your educational audiologist to determine if these parts must be obtained through your implant center or if they are available through the school system. If your child's school does not have an audiologist, be sure to discuss this with your implant center.

Radiology Procedures

Because of the internal magnet in the receiver-stimulator, magnetic resonance imaging (MRI) procedures may need to be modified. Currently, one device is compatible with a low strength MRI. The other two devices have removable magnets, which require a minor surgical procedure to "pop out" the magnet, and this can then easily be replaced in the receiver-stimulator after the MRI is completed. Even with these removable magnets, full strength MRI is not recommended. If your child is in need of these procedures, discussing options with your physicians would be an important consideration when choosing an implant system.

Testing the Implant after Insertion

It is possible to test the implant system immediately after insertion to see if it is appropriately positioned and functioning. Verification that the implant is working correctly utilizes the *electrical compound action potential* (ECAP). The ECAP is an electrical signal generated when the cochlear nerve transmits a signal. Consequently, when an ECAP is identified following electrical stimulation, it means that the nerve itself has been stimulated and information is being sent to the brain. A present acoustic nerve action potential means that your child is highly likely to be able to perceive stimulation through the implant.

An absent ECAP requires that the audiologist look very carefully at the system to determine the reason for the absence of the action potential. Each implant manufacturer provides a system to obtain a response from the auditory nerve derived from electrical stimulation. This procedure can be performed in the operating room during surgery or at any appointment after surgery when your child sees the audiologist for routine follow-up care. The presence of the ECAP at the time of surgery is very reassuring to parents who may be nervous about the possibility of implant failure. Other information may be needed to verify functionality of the system, such as behavioral results, cortical evoked potentials, or electrical stapedial reflex thresholds (ESRT).

Recording the compound action potential has become a quick, non-invasive procedure. It is objective and requires very little cooperation by the child. In addition to confirming that the CI is providing stimulation, the ECAP can also help to estimate programming parameters and can provide a baseline for observing changes in neural response over time. Cochlear Corporation calls its ECAP system Neural Response Telemetry (NRT). Advanced Bionics Corporation calls its ECAP system Neural Response Imaging (NRI), and Med-El calls its ECAP system Auditory Nerve Response Telemetry (ART).

Batteries

Batteries can be one of the most costly parts of the device. Although rechargeable batteries are available from all three manufacturers, they are not available for all wearing options. It is important to make sure the battery option you want to use is available for the wearing option you have chosen. If your child is going to use an FM system at school, find out if the rechargeable battery option can be used at the same time.

Battery life varies between companies and devices. Your child's programs will also affect battery life.

Cochlear Implant Manufacturers

Current Advanced Bionics Corporation Products

Advanced Bionics currently has two completely different speech processors available for patients. The Platinum Series Sound Processor

(PSP) body-worn device is worn on a harness or a belt clip. It is available for small children, who are not able to support a device on the ear, or elderly patients who may have some vision or dexterity issues. The microphone is integrated into the headpiece and the device controls are large and easy to see. There is a visual and auditory alarm that can be programmed to indicate problems. There are two different battery options, including rechargeable proprietary Lithium Ion batteries or AA batteries. The Intellilink safety feature allows a speech processor to only stimulate a single, designated CI. This keeps children with bilateral CIs from accidentally switching devices and being stimulated.

Advanced Bionics' BTE device is called the Harmony. It has a built-in indicator light to enable monitoring of the system. The program switch allows the user to switch between up to three programs. There is a volume control that can be disabled. There are two different sizes of proprietary rechargeable batteries that allow for up to a full day of power. They also have the option of interchangeable earhooks that can be added for use with different accessories.

Advanced Bionics' internal device is the HiRes 90K CI. The device uses 16 electrodes, which Advanced Bionics reports are designed for consistent signal generation and precise information delivery. The newest sound processing option from Advanced Bionics is HiRes Fidelity 120. It reports that it is designed to help with listening in noisy situations and to improve the sound quality when listening to music. With this technology, they use current steering technology to increase spectral resolution from as few as 12 to 22 spectral bands to as many as 120 spectral bands. Currently, this is only approved in the United States by the Food and Drug Administration for use with adults.

Current Cochlear Corporation Products

Cochlear Corporation's newest implant system is the Nucleus Freedom system. The Freedom Sound Processor can be worn as a BTE unit, as a Babyworn unit, or as a body-worn unit. All three wearing options have an LCD panel that gives certain information about the implant system such as sensitivity, telecoil, volume, battery level, and a program display. The main processing module/speech processor can be attached to different parts, which make up the three wearing options. For the Freedom BTE, the speech processor is attached to a BTE controller/battery pack, which is worn completely behind the ear. The Freedom BTE controller comes in a two- and three-battery controller. Some patients are not able to utilize the Freedom mini-BTE battery pack (controller) because of the power requirements of their program. Talk to your CI audiologist about what is best for your child. The Babyworn option has a cable that separates the speech processor from the BTE battery pack, so that the BTE battery pack can be pinned to a shirt. There is a Retention Case that protects the battery pack and has different methods of pinning or attaching the processing unit to the child's clothing. The body-worn option has a Bodyworn Controller User Interface, which is connected to the speech processor by a cable. The Bodyworn Controller User Interface has the same LCD screen as the BTE controller. Centers that use a two-processor system allow the patient to choose two of the battery packs. This is based on patient preference.

There are several electrode arrays in the Nucleus Freedom system. The most common electrode array is the Contour Advance. This electrode array has 22 electrodes and Cochlear Corporation indicates that it is designed for lifetime use, with electronics capable of compatibility with future equipment and software upgrades. This electrode array is called a perimodiolar electrode, because the array is housed in material that flexes the electrode around the bends in the cochlea, keeping the electrodes as close as possible to the nerve fibers that it is stimulating. Also available with the Freedom system is a straight electrode array, used in certain medical situations to be determined by the surgeon. Cochlear Corporation has the Nucleus Double Array, which is used when full insertion of the standard array is not possible, such as in cases where the cause of the hearing loss is meningitis.

Another feature of the Nucleus Freedom system is SmartSound. This feature adds several automatic and user controlled features to improve a user's performance in background noise. SmartSound includes an Autosensitivity control, which Cochlear Corporation indicates is designed to automatically prevent background noise from becoming too loud. Another feature of SmartSound is Whisper. This feature uses compression to increase a listener's ability to hear softer sounds. Still another feature is ADRO, which is an automatically adjusting algorithm designed to remove unwanted sound and enhance wanted sounds. Finally, the last feature of SmartSound is a feature called Beam. Beam reduces the microphone input from the rear and sides of the listener, effectively emphasizing inputs from the front.

Current Med-El Corporation Products

Med-El has the Opus 1 and Opus 2 speech processor systems, with the smallest and lightest speech processor system on the market. The company utilizes a modular design that allows patients to wear their speech processor in five different wearing options. The Opus 1 speech processor has two different switches that control the programs and volumes. There is also a sensitivity knob and a status light that indicates the need for troubleshooting. The Opus 2 speech processor has a streamlined design, without switches or knobs. It utilizes a remote control for changing features. This will allow patients to change programs, volume, and sensitivity without having to touch their device. Patients will receive the speech processor with different battery packs that can be changed out based on the patient's lifestyle and needs. The Baby BTE allows the patient to wear the processor and the straight battery pack pinned to the shoulder with a long cord connecting to the coil. This works best for infants and small children who are not ready or able to wear the processor behind their ear. The Children's Battery Pack allows patients to wear the processor on the ear and the battery pack pinned to the shoulder. This is a great transition option for children. The Angled Battery Pack and the Straight Battery Pack are both worn behind the ear. Both are options that can be utilized based on patient preference. The Remote Battery Pack is worn with the speech processor on the ear and the battery pack at the waist. The Opus 2 speech processor uses both proprietary rechargeable and disposable batteries. All battery packs come in the patient kit, allowing flexibility in your wearing option.

Med-El offers two different implants that utilize their I^{100} electronics platform. These are the SONATA^{100} CI and the PULSAR^{100} CI. Med-El reports that both implants allow a greater amount of information to be processed while keeping energy requirements to a minimum. The Med-El electrode uses 24 electrodes arranged as 12 twin surfaces. The SONATA^{100} is the lightest titanium CI on the market, whereas the PULSAR^{100} is a compact ceramic device. The Med-El Standard Electrode Array provides the deepest insertion and is the most commonly used Med-El array. The Medium Electrode Array may be used when a deep insertion is not possible, the Compressed Electrode Array may be used in the case of ossification or cochlear malformations, and the Split Electrode Array may be used in the case of severe ossification.

The Med-El speech processors allow for two different coding strategies. These are the Fine Structure Processing (FSP) coding strategy and high definition continuous interleaved sampling (HD-CIS). They both utilize an Adaptive Sound Window that allows for an extended input dynamic range, helping the patient to hear soft sounds while keeping loud sounds comfortable. Med-El believes this also helps patients hear the wide range of music, allowing them to enjoy the complexity of it.

Company-specific information presented in this section was provided by each manufacturer. Much of the information is available on their Web sites, and the Web site addresses can be found in the Resources section of this book.

CIs have progressed from early products that offered very little chance for their recipients to use electrical stimulation for language learning to advanced products now offering the potential for normal language development in appropriately selected recipients. Research and development will continue to offer new technologies, with improved outcomes sure to follow. The selection of the implant system is a highly personal decision that should be based upon the needs of the child and the family. Discussing this with other CI families is often useful in determining which system might be right for your child. You should also seek the professional advice of your implant team to assist in choosing the implant device likely to provide the best results.

Reference

Brown, C. J. (2003). The electrically evoked whole nerve action potential. In H. E. Cullington (Ed.), *Cochlear implants: Objective measures* (pp. 96–129). London: Whurr.

Chute, P. M., & Nevins, M. E. (2002). *The parents' guide to cochlear implants.* Washington, DC: Gallaudet University Press.

Patrick, J. F., Seligman, P. M., & Clark, G. M. (1997). Engineering. In G. M. Clark, R. S. C. Cowan, & R. C. Dowell (Eds.), *Cochlear implantation for infants and children: Advances* (pp. 125–146). San Diego, CA: Singular.

Rance, G., & Dowell, R. C. (1997). Speech processor programming. In G. M. Clark, R. S. C. Cowan, & R. C. Dowell (Eds.), *Cochlear implantation for infants and children: Advances* (pp. 147–170). San Diego, CA: Singular.

Villchur, E. (2000). *Acoustics for audiologists.* San Diego, CA: Singular.

Wilson, B. S. (2006). Speech processing strategies. In H. R. Cooper & L. C. Craddock (Eds.), *Cochlear implants: A practical guide* (pp. 21–69). London: Whurr.

Chapter 6

Cochlear Implant Surgery

By Peter S. Roland

The Cochlear Implant Surgical Process

Why Surgery?

The operation that is required to place a cochlear implant (CI) is an appropriate cause of concern for both you and your child. An operation is necessary because a CI works by stimulating the cochlear nerve directly. In order to do so, the CI electrode array must be placed as close as possible to the cochlear nerve. The nerve endings of the cochlea lie within a coiled tube called the cochlear duct. This is a big advantage for CI surgery because it allows the electrodes to be placed very close to the ends of the cochlear nerve simply by inserting the electrode array into this coiled cochlear duct. The cochlea lies within the skull base just behind the eardrum. A pin, approximately 2 inches in length, passed along the ear canal and through the eardrum, would stop when it came to rest against the cochlea. Theoretically, therefore, one way to place a CI would be to put the electrode under the skin in the ear canal and through the eardrum. Electrodes are rarely placed in the ear canal because electrodes in the ear canal tend to erode through the skin and become exposed. Exposure in the open ear canal has led to infection that is difficult to eradicate and requires implant removal. Consequently, CI electrode arrays are placed by putting them through the mastoid cavity behind the ear canal.

It takes a surgeon about an hour to an hour and a half to perform the operation required to place the implant. An additional half hour is required at the beginning and the end of the operation in order to put your child to sleep and then wake her up. Consequently, it is 2 to 3 hours between the time a patient enters the operating area and the time she arrives in the recovery room. Complicated or difficult cases may take longer.

Day Surgery and Overnight Stays

Surgery for cochlear implantation is frequently performed as a day surgery procedure. Patients arrive at the hospital during the day, have the operation, and then leave that same day without spending the night in the hospital. This has now been evaluated in the scientific literature and has been determined to be quite safe. Even though it's safe, you may feel pretty uncomfortable going home with your child only a few hours after a general anesthetic and a surgical procedure. You may feel uncomfortable with the idea of caring for someone who has been put to sleep and awakened so recently. This is especially true if the operation has occurred late in the day or if you live several hours from the hospital. The experience of thousands of patients, however, confirms that day surgery is safe and that individuals who have had their operations as day surgery procedures are not placed at greater risk than individuals who spend the night in the hospital.

Although day surgery is appropriate for most healthy individuals, children with certain medical conditions have a slightly higher risk of complications after general anesthesia. If the condition is temporary, then the operation is often deferred. A cold is a good example of such a condition. An upper respiratory infection (a cold) does increase the risk of anesthesia, though only very slightly. Even though the increased risk is slight, the concern for patient safety among anesthesiologists and surgeons is such that non-emergency operations are deferred until the patient is healthy. If the medical condition cannot be entirely eliminated, then the attempt is made to improve the condition before the operation is performed and the patient is asked to spend the night in the hospital to make sure the risk of complications is minimized. Individuals with heart disease or lung conditions (like asthma or COPD), for example, fall into the latter category. If your child has severe sleep apnea, the operation is usually performed in an inpatient setting and you are asked to spend the night after surgery. Anesthesiologists and surgeons can be relied upon to know when an individual's underlying medical condition makes staying overnight in the hospital the safest option.

Medical Considerations

Ear Tubes

Many children who are candidates for cochlear implantation have ear tubes. These tubes are placed through the eardrum in order to allow fluid to escape and air to enter the middle ear behind the eardrum. Tubes reduce the incidence of middle ear infections. The placement of tubes into the eardrum is now the most common operation in the United States, so many children have tubes at the time the operation is performed. Surgeons differ a little bit on how they handle children with ear tubes. Most surgeons are comfortable performing the procedure even though tubes are in the eardrum. Some surgeons remove the tube at the time the CI is placed; other surgeons leave the tube in position and allow it to be pushed out of the eardrum naturally over the next several weeks or months.

Infections

Infection of the CI wound is a serious complication of CI surgery. Fortunately, it is uncommon. It occurs in only 1 to 2% of CI recipients. Sometimes, such infections can be managed with the use of antibiotics, but sometimes they cannot. When an infection does not respond to postoperative antibiotics, then the CI needs to be removed and the process has to start all over again. Therefore, it's important to do everything possible to eliminate the risk of postoperative infection. The use of rigorous sterile technique in the operating room is the most important method of eliminating infections. This includes the use of sterilized instruments, good hand washing by operating room personnel, and the use of antiseptics to eliminate skin bacteria. Antibiotics are given just before the skin incision and continue for about 24 hours following surgery. Several modern antibiotics last 24 hours after being given intravenously, and consequently, no antibiotics need to be taken by mouth after the operation. Studies have shown that using antibiotics for more than 24 hours after the operation *does not* reduce the risk of surgical infection; thus, it is not necessary to take antibiotics for days after the operation.

It is now known that shaving hair in the area of the incision is not necessary to prevent infection. Removing small amounts of hair does make closing the incision easier, so small amounts of hair are sometimes removed from behind the ear as part of the operation. Many surgeons, however, no longer shave any hair at all.

The Surgical Procedure

General Anesthesia

General anesthesia is almost universally utilized for CI surgery. Over the past 50 years, a tremendous amount of effort has gone into making general anesthesia safe. Years of training beyond medical school are required to become a board certified anesthesiologist. Additional training is required to become a fellowship trained and board certified pediatric anesthesiologist. A great deal of this training is directed toward ensuring patient safety and minimizing risks and complications. Modern anesthetics are much safer than earlier anesthetics, and contemporary anesthetic techniques utilize monitoring equipment that continuously assesses how the patient is doing. Pulse, blood pressure, and respiratory rate are all monitored throughout the operation. The anesthesiologist is aware at all times of how much oxygen the patient is receiving and how much carbon dioxide she is exhaling. It is possible, when necessary, to know the exact oxygen content of the patient's blood continuously throughout the operation. Because of this, the risk of serious complications is very low in healthy individuals. Even children with serious medical conditions, including advanced heart and lung disease, can be put to sleep and awakened safely (Figure 6–1).

Even though anesthesia is statistically very safe, it is quite frightening for many parents. This is partly because general anesthesia is a risk you are not accustomed to. Statistically, the risk of being involved in a serious car accident each time you take a drive in your automo-

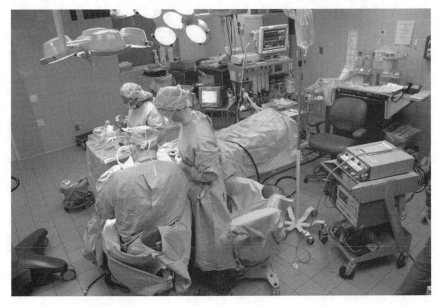

Figure 6–1. This is how the operating room is set up for cochlear implant surgery. The scrub nurse is usually across the table from the surgeon. The room stays well lit until the microscope is brought into use.

bile is about the same as the risk of serious complication from general anesthesia if you are healthy. However, the risks associated with driving are ones we are accustomed to and are therefore less frightening.

Incisions

The surgical incisions used to place a CI have been refined and greatly reduced in size over the last 10 to 15 years. Relatively large U-shaped incisions were used for many years, but it is now common for the incision to be no longer than a couple of inches. The incision is placed about a finger width behind the crease formed where the external ear meets the scalp skin (Figure 6-2). The exact length of the incision varies a little bit between one surgeon and another and is partially determined by the type of CI placed. Some types of CIs require a slightly longer incision than others (Figure 6-3).

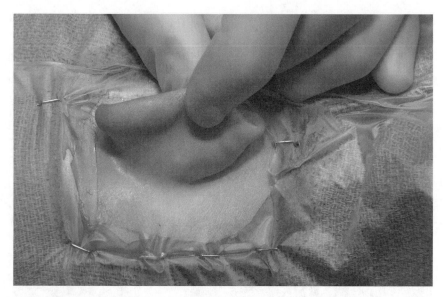

Figure 6–2. After the ear and surrounding scalp have been prepared with antiseptic solution, an incision is planned about a finger breadth behind the attachment of the external ear.

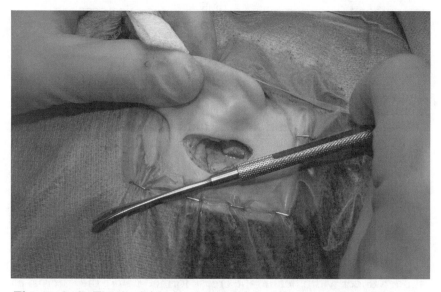

Figure 6–3. The incision is about 1½ to 2 inches long. In this picture, next to the incision, you can see the instrument (a periosteal elevator) that will be used to create the pocket that holds the stimulator-receiver.

Exposure of the Middle Ear

Once the incision has been made, the bone behind the external ear is identified. The outside layer of this bone is removed to expose the air cells of the mastoid itself (Figure 6-4). The mastoid bone is not solid: it consists of a honeycomb of air cells, so that the normal mastoid is about 90% air and less than 10% bone. These air cells are removed to provide access to the middle ear (Figure 6-5). What was once 90% air is turned into a cavity that is 100% air. The purpose of the mastoid, insofar as it can be determined, is to function as an air reservoir for the middle ear. Because of this, it is believed that removing the mastoid air cells, if anything, improves its function. Once these air cells are removed, the middle ear can be approached from behind without disturbing the eardrum (Figure 6-6). In order to do so, it is necessary to pass very close to the facial nerve. Injury to the facial nerve is one of

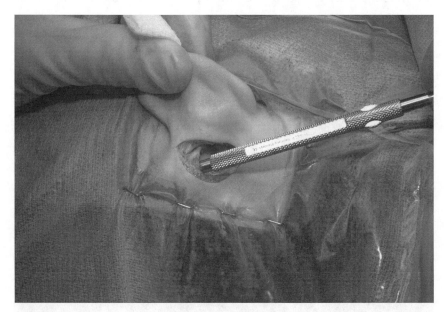

Figure 6–4. The elevator is in position beneath the soft tissues on the bone of the skull. This is how the "pocket" is created that will hold the stimulator-receiver. By comparing this picture with Figure 6–3, you can get an idea of how deep the pocket is. This also shows you the direction in which the pocket is created.

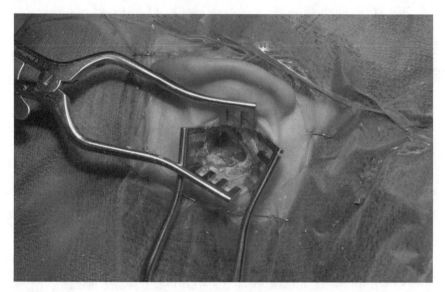

Figure 6–5. After the soft tissue pocket has been created to house the stimulator-receiver, a surgical burr is used to open up the mastoid cavity. This is what the open mastoid cavity looks like.

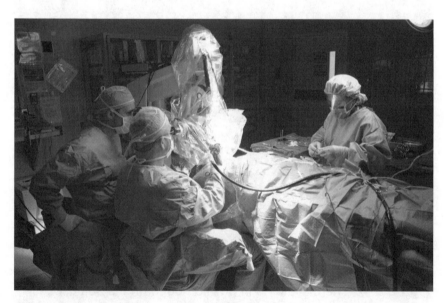

Figure 6–6. Once the mastoid cavity has been created, a microscope is brought into use. When the microscope is utilized, most of the lights in the operating room are turned off. This makes it easier to see detail through the microscope.

the most feared risks of CI surgery because injury to the nerve results in paralysis of that side of the face. Paralysis of the face is considered unsightly and, therefore, great efforts are taken to make sure that injury to the facial nerve does not occur. Experienced surgeons understand the anatomy of the facial nerve well and use that knowledge to make sure the facial nerve is not damaged. Special facial nerve monitors are used during the operation that tell the surgeon if he gets close to the facial nerve. While the use of facial nerve monitors does not guarantee that the facial nerve will escape injury, it minimizes the risk. Facial nerve monitors are almost universally utilized during CI surgery. Overall, injury to the facial nerve occurs in less than 1% of individuals receiving CIs, and for many experienced surgeons, the risk is very much lower. Many surgeons have performed hundreds upon hundreds of CIs with no permanent facial nerve injuries. Occasionally, the facial nerve is bruised and temporary paralysis results. In such circumstances, the facial nerve recovers completely within a matter of weeks or months.

Insertion of Electrode Array and Receiver

Once the middle ear is exposed from behind, a small hole is made into the cochlea. This allows access to the cochlear duct. Once this access has been achieved, the CI electrode array is slid into the cochlea. The electrodes come to rest within a 10th of an inch or less of the ends of the cochlear nerve. This allows very small currents to effectively stimulate the cochlear nerve and produce hearing.

Either just before or just after the electrode is placed, the stimulator-receiver must be placed beneath the skin behind the ear. A small pocket under the skin is made behind the incision to accommodate the stimulator–receiver. Traditionally, a "bone bed" was created to accommodate the stimulator-receiver. A bone bed is created by removing the bone of the skull in the exact shape of the CI stimulator-receiver (Figure 6-7, Figure 6-8, Figure 6-9, and Figure 6-10). The CI stimulator-receiver then fits into this bony depression in the skull designed to accommodate it. In adults, the bone is relatively thick— a quarter of an inch or more. Thus, one can make a shallow bone bed and still leave bone between the CI stimulator-receiver and the lining of the brain, called the dura mater. However, in small children, the bone is only a 10th of an inch thick. Removing bone to accommodate the

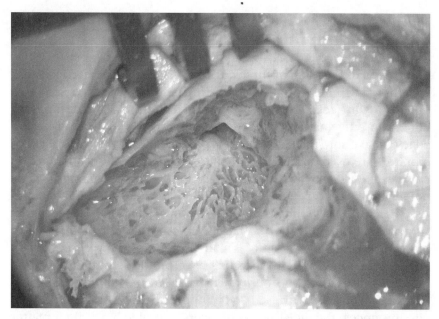

Figure 6–7. This is a view of the mastoid cavity using the microscope. None of the microsurgical drilling has yet been done.

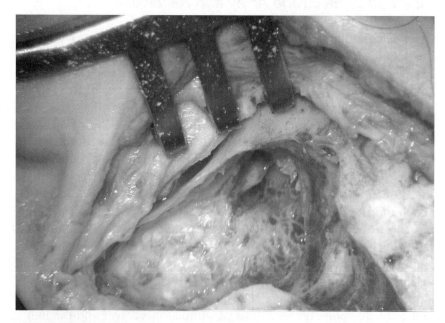

Figure 6–8. The facial recess has been started. You can see what it looks like at completion in Figure 6–10.

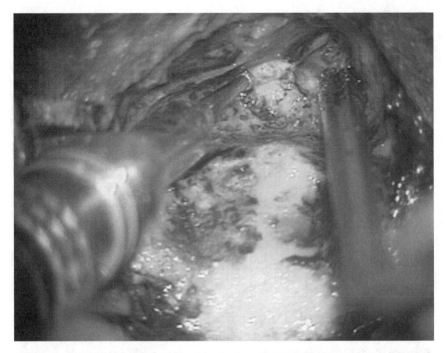

Figure 6–9. A very small burr can be seen opening up the facial recess. The instrument to the right is a combined suction-irrigator —water comes out continuously from the lower tube and is then removed by suction through the upper tube.

stimulator-receiver exposes the lining of the brain (the dura mater), and sometimes the lining of the brain is pushed inward when the CI stimulator-receiver is placed into the bone bed. This is potentially dangerous. Drilling the bone bed has resulted in spinal fluid leaks and serious blood clots. Some surgeons view this as the most dangerous part of the operation and no longer drill a bone bed. When a bone bed is not drilled, the CI sometimes creates a little lump that can be seen and felt in the skin behind the ear. This is usually not visible from a distance because it is covered by hair. Some surgeons elect to accept this lumpiness in order to make the operation safer. Similarly, it has been traditional to drill holes into the bone in order to pass sutures over the stimulator-receiver and secure it tightly to the underlying bone. In order to do so, a drill must be utilized to drill a hole into the bone. When this is done, the drill must be aimed directly toward the

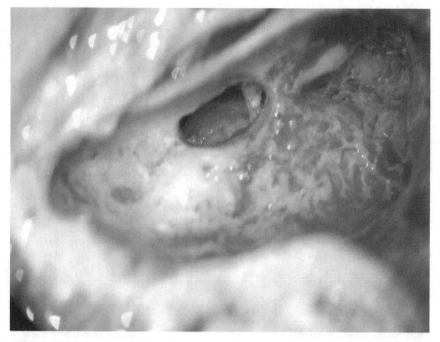

Figure 6–10. The facial recess dissection is completed. You can see the inculo-stapedeal joint through the recess and the bone of the cochlea beneath it.

brain. If the drill goes even a little too deeply, it can penetrate the lining of the brain and create a cerebrospinal fluid leak or a blood clot inside the skull. Again, some surgeons no longer drill holes to secure the stimulator-receiver to the underlying bone because they believe that it is safer not to do so. When a bed and drill holes are omitted, there is some risk of the CI moving. This can, on rare occasions, cause the CI to fail because movement results in repetitive bending of the wires that leads to breakage; or, if the implant moves a lot, it can pull the electrode array out of the cochlea. When this occurs, the implant must be replaced.

Once the stimulator-receiver has been placed underneath the skin and the electrode array has been inserted into the cochlea, a small piece of tissue is wrapped around the electrode array to seal the opening into the cochlea (Figure 6–11, Figure 6–12). This prevents

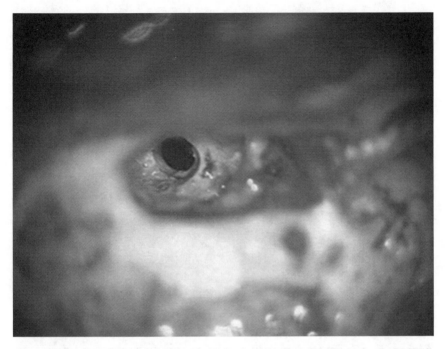

Figure 6–11. The cochleostomy has been made. This is the black hole that can be seen through the facial recess. The cochlear implant electrode array will be carefully threaded through this opening into the cochlea.

infection from getting into the cochlea. Infection within the cochlea can lead to meningitis. The incision is then closed and a dressing is placed. The child is awakened in the recovery room and either sent home with you a few hours later or, if your child's underlying medical condition requires it, you will be asked to stay in the hospital overnight.

After Surgery

The dressing is usually left on at least overnight (Figure 6-13). Some surgeons prefer to leave it on a little longer. The dressing often includes gauze pads over the incision. This makes the dressing lumpy and uncomfortable. Because the dressing is a little uncomfortable, your

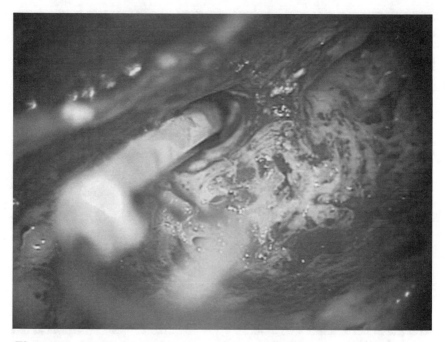

Figure 6–12. The cochlear implant electrode array has been successfully threaded into the cochlea. The cochlear implant operation will be completed once the stimulator-receiver has been placed into the soft tissue pocket behind the incision. The incision will then be sown up.

child will be happy when the dressing is removed. The day following CI surgery, recipients can generally engage in all activities except swimming and very active physical movement. Children should be encouraged to avoid very strenuous activities like tumbling, wrestling, soccer, and other contact sports for a few days after the operation.

Following surgery, patients can eat anything they want but should start with a light meal first. If the light meal is tolerated, then a heavier meal can be taken. The wound is achy and painful for about 24 to 48 hours. For the first 24 to 36 hours, a mild narcotic pain medicine should be utilized—usually one with codeine. After 36 to 48 hours, nonnarcotic pain medicines like Tylenol, Aleve, and Motrin are often sufficient. When they provide adequate pain control, nonnarcotic medicines are preferred because they lack the side effects of nausea, vomiting, constipation, and dizziness. The wound generally stops

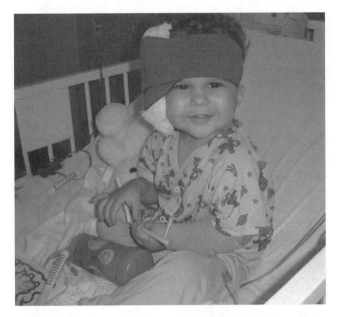

Figure 6–13. Jared, pictured here in the recovery room after surgery, received a unilateral cochlear implant for his right ear.

hurting after 36 to 48 hours but remains tender to touch for several more days.

Some slight swelling behind the ear can be expected. The swelling is often sufficient to push the ear forward. Many parents worry that the ear will not grow back to its normal position, but it almost always does. Scabs can form over the incision. Scab formation is normal and no effort should be made to remove the scab. The wound can be cleaned with hydrogen peroxide, and an antibiotic ointment can be placed on the wound if desired, but this is not necessary. A small amount of bleeding from the wound is common in the first 24 to 36 hours and is not anything to worry about. More extensive bleeding should be reported to the operating surgeon.

Bruising behind the ear is fairly common. Occasionally, bruising will develop in front of the ear and can produce a "black eye." The black eye will disappear in a week or two.

Surgeons differ a little bit in how long they ask patients to wait before showering or bathing. Many surgeons permit showering and bathing after 24 to 48 hours. Wounds generally seal to bacteria over that period of time. Drainage from the ear canal is not typical but does occur in some circumstances. Individuals who have had a tube in place at the time of the CI placement will generally have some draining from the ear canal for up to 48 to 72 hours after the operation. Occasionally, during placement of the CI, either the ear canal skin or the eardrum will be injured, and fluid can come out of the ear canal even though no tube was in position at the time of the operation. If drainage from the ear occurs, it should be reported to the operating surgeon. Often antibiotic drops to prevent infection will be prescribed. The drops should be placed into the ear canal two to three times per day until the drainage stops.

Complications

Dizziness and Imbalance

Table 6–1 lists some uncommon risks associated with CI surgery. Imbalance and dizziness sometimes occur after CI placement. It usually lasts no more than 36 to 48 hours. Dizziness can be the result of placing the electrode array into the cochlea, the result of anesthesia, a side effect of codeine-containing pain medication, or a combination of all of these factors. If it lasts longer than 48 hours, the operating surgeon should be notified.

Table 6–1. Risks associated with cochlear implantation

The following risks are considered to have a low occurrence rate:

- The presence of the internal component may cause a bump behind your ear.

- The implant may cause irritation, inflammation, or breakdown of the skin around the area of the internal component.

- Your body may reject the device or the device may move to a position in your ear that is not functional.

Table 6–1. *continued*

- The operation may fail, perhaps requiring removal of the device.

- The device may fail requiring its removal and replacement. When parts of the internal device fail, it may result in fewer electrodes available for programming or may result in the perception of uncomfortably loud sounds.

- When the implant is activated, you may experience facial nerve stimulation or involuntary facial movement.

- You may experience numbness or stiffness around the surgically implanted ear. This may continue for 4 to 6 months following surgery.

- Neck pain may continue for several weeks after the surgery.

- There is a possibility that facial nerve paralysis or weakness of a temporary or permanent nature may occur after the surgery.

- You may experience taste disturbance or mouth dryness for a minimal, prolonged, or indefinite period of time.

- You may experience leaking of inner ear or spinal fluid into the surgical site. Surgery may be required to repair this and this may also lead to meningitis.

- The incidence of meningitis in cochlear implant recipients, while low, may be higher than in individuals who have not received a cochlear implant. Vaccination against the bacteria pneumococcus may significantly reduce the risk of meningitis and is highly recommended for both adult and pediatric recipients.

- Dizziness or unsteadiness may occur immediately following the surgery. Unsteadiness may persist for several weeks after the surgery, but prolonged dizziness is rare.

- Tinnitus or ringing in the ear may be experienced following surgery. This is often temporary but can be permanent.

- The external components of the implant system may cause skin reactions.

It is considered highly likely that the following will happen:

- Any residual hearing that you had before the surgery will be destroyed.

Facial Nerve Weakness

Occasionally, mild compression or bruising of the facial nerve results in facial weakness, developing hours or even several days after the operation. This is generally nothing to worry about; the facial nerve will recover over a period of a week to a couple of months. However, it should be immediately reported to the operating surgeon because most surgeons will prescribe a short course of steroids to reduce facial nerve swelling and speed up recovery.

The nerve that provides taste to the front part of half of the tongue passes through the middle ear. This nerve can be stretched during the CI operation. When the nerve is stretched, it produces a funny metallic taste in the mouth. This is similar to the metallic taste that is often associated with an upper respiratory infection or cold. This alteration of taste usually disappears after several days or a couple of weeks. If this small nerve providing taste, called the chorda tympani nerve, is cut, as is occasionally necessary to place the implant, then taste from one fourth of the tongue will be permanently absent.

Infection

Wound infection is a serious complication. It usually becomes apparent 24 to 48 hours after the operation but sometimes does not become apparent for several days. Signs of developing infection can include increasing rather than decreasing pain, redness of the skin, oozing of a milky, white, pus-like material from the incision, and occasionally fever. Again, anything suggesting infection should be reported immediately to the operating surgeon.

When identified early, infections around an implant can sometimes be successfully treated without removing the implant. Implant removal, however, is sometimes necessary to eradicate the infection. If an implant has been removed because of infection, it can usually be replaced 6 to 8 weeks later. Very rarely, meningitis follows placement of a CI. This is most likely to occur in individuals who have congenital malformations of the inner ear. Since preoperative imaging—either a CT scan or an MRI—is usually performed prior to CI placement, patients and surgeons are aware that such a malformation exists prior to placing the implant. Anything suggesting meningitis should be reported to the surgeon immediately. Symptoms of meningitis include undue sleepiness or disorientation, a stiff neck, severe headache, and fever over 101°. Table 6–2 lists reasons to contact your surgeon after surgery.

Spinal Fluid Leaks

Occasionally, spinal fluid leaks from the wound or into the middle ear and down the throat. This can occur because the lining of the brain (the dura mater) has been injured as a result of drilling the bed or suture holes for the stimulator-receiver or because a congenital malformation connects the cochlea itself with the spinal fluid surrounding the brain. Spinal fluid leaks appear as clear, watery fluid coming from the wound, the ear canal, or the nose. It should be immediately reported to the operating surgeon.

There are two ways of managing a spinal fluid leak. It can be managed with a spinal drain. A spinal drain is a thin, flexible plastic tube placed low in the back. It diverts spinal fluid by removing it through the spinal drain. This reduces the pressure of spinal fluid passing into the wound and allows the wound to heal and seal the spinal fluid leak. When spinal drainage is utilized, it usually requires

Table 6–2. Reasons to contact the operating surgeon after surgery

- Wound infection:
  - Increasing pain
  - Redness of skin
  - Oozing of pus-like material from incision
  - Fever
- Meningitis symptoms:
  - Fever over 101°
  - Undue sleepiness or disorientation
  - Stiff neck
- Spinal fluid leaks:
  - Clear, watery fluid from the wound, ear canal, nose

3 to 5 days for it to work. Your child must be in the hospital during this time. An alternative way of managing a spinal fluid leak is to go back to the operating room and surgically repair the area from which the spinal fluid is leaking. This requires an additional operation; however, patients can often go home the following day. The presence of a spinal fluid leak increases the risk of meningitis, although very few patients with spinal fluid leaks actually develop meningitis. This is a serious condition and a suspicion of spinal fluid leak should be reported immediately to the operating surgeon.

Fortunately, CI surgery is uneventful for most recipients. The operation usually proceeds without difficulty and without complications and your child is back to her usual activity level in a couple of days. It is important to remember that the CI will not produce hearing until the CI is activated and the external portions of the CI are fitted to the implanted stimulator-receiver. Programming of the device and placement of the external portions occur somewhere between a day and 3 weeks following CI surgery. How long after the operation the implant is actually activated varies from center to center.

The Brothers' Story

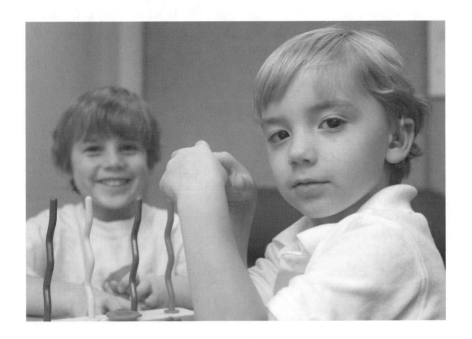

We were, of course, quite upset when John was diagnosed with a hearing loss. However, we had been suspecting he had some hearing issues for several months, so it wasn't a complete surprise. We were surprised though by how severe his hearing loss was (profound). At the time we were pretty ignorant about hearing loss and had no idea what to do. My husband and I are both practical people, so our immediate response was, "We will fix the problem—whatever it takes." I thought there must be some surgery or procedure that could be done to correct his hearing. I don't think I fully understood the severity and permanence of the loss.

The night we found out about the hearing loss, the first thing we did was go home and get on-line and start researching the topic of hearing loss. We read extensively on the subject. We also talked to our pediatrician, our pediatric ENT, and friends and family, and we found two couples who also had children with hearing loss. We contacted them and started gaining information. We got referrals to a cochlear implant physician and an auditory verbal therapist. We made appointments and got started right away in helping John to hear.

It was scary in the beginning because we had no idea how to begin helping John with his hearing, and we knew that every week that went by he was getting further and further behind with his listening and speaking. So we felt under pressure to do something. We just trusted all the other parents, doctors, audiologists, and therapists and hoped we were doing the right things for our son! It looks now like we did the right things.

When our next son, Todd, was born, we had his hearing tested early on. Sure enough, he also had a profound hearing loss, just like John. We were surprised and disappointed but not shocked, because we already had one son with a hearing loss. I felt we were repeating the entire process! However, this time, we were very informed and knew just what to do.

John will enter mainstream kindergarten in the fall at our neighborhood school and Todd attends a mainstream preschool program.

—Anne McPherson, mother of John and Todd

Chapter 7

Initial Stimulation and MAPping: What to Expect

By Andrea D. Warner-Czyz

You have waited for this moment to arrive, when your child will enter or reenter the world of hearing. How exciting that your child will hear your voice, her own voice, and environmental sounds! Hearing sounds will be a big change from the silent world your child knows and will transform how you interact with your child. This change often generates a range of emotions including anticipation, anxiety, apprehension, doubt, and excitement for both you and your child.

To prepare for the moment when your child begins to hear, you need to know what to expect as your child goes through the cochlear implant (CI) process. The first session with the audiologist after your child's surgery has two primary goals: (a) to introduce your child to sound with the CI and (b) to familiarize both you and your child to the device's external equipment. Because this is the first time that the audiologist stimulates, or turns on, the CI, it is often called the *initial stimulation*. It may also be called the CI activation, device hookup, or device switch-on.

The initial stimulation appointment often spans a 2-day period, with sessions lasting between 1½ and 4 hours each day. The appointment will be scheduled 2 to 4 weeks after your child's surgery to allow time for the surgical incision to heal and for the swelling to decrease. The healed incision will decrease discomfort of the skin and tissues and the reduced swelling will provide better access to the magnetic receiver implanted behind your child's ear. Both are important to make sure your child has a positive, comfortable experience when the external equipment is connected. Your physician must give you medical clearance before the initial stimulation appointment can occur. Children under 3 years of age are usually scheduled with two audiologists so that one can program your child's CI while the other observes your child's responses to sound. Using two audiologists will yield the best results because it highlights the importance of making your child the focus of this appointment.

The initial stimulation session centers on introducing your child to sound with the CI. The settings of the CI device, called the *MAP*, will be the starting point of your child's hearing experience. The first goal of this initial MAP is not to provide perfect hearing, but to serve as the baseline for future MAPs. Remember that your child has not listened to sound in a while (or maybe not at all), so early hearing with the CI will be like that of a newborn baby. Just like an infant, though, your child gradually will adapt to the world of hearing and sound over time. This first MAP—your child's first experience with sound—is a very important step to your child's success with the CI device.

The second goal of the initial appointment is to teach you and your child to operate, manipulate, and maintain the equipment. It is crucial that you learn to care for your child's CI equipment and know what to do if it breaks. The manufacturer and your audiologist will give you brochures about your child's CI equipment. This chapter focuses on the initial stimulation and future programming of your child's CI.

The basic goals of the initial appointment, introduction to sound and the CI device, do not cover the strong emotions you will feel during this time. It is possible that because of these emotions, you may not retain everything that the audiologist tells you. You will be able to learn this material from brochures and DVDs and from your audiologist, who will be available for any questions or concerns that arise. Remember that your child should be the center of attention during the initial stimulation appointment. It might help to let siblings and extended family stay at home so that you can focus on the child who is receiving the CI. His first experience with sound influences future success, so work with the audiologists to make it a positive experience. The more involved you are—and the more you show your child that you accept this new device—the better the chance that your child will accept it as well. Your child will follow your lead to accept the CI.

What can you do to prepare your child for what he is about to experience? What do you need to know about the initial stimulation of your child's CI? First, you need to know what to expect from your audiologist. Second, you need to know what to expect from your child. Third, you need to know what to expect from yourself.

What to Expect from Your Audiologist

Before we talk about what happens at the initial stimulation appointment with your audiologist, let's review the parts of the CI and how these parts work together. There are two major portions of the CI device: the external and internal parts.

The *external* part of the device includes a battery supply, microphone, speech processor, cable, and transmission coil. The *battery supply* provides electric energy to the external part of the device. A small *microphone* collects sound and sends it to the speech processor. The *speech processor* digitizes the sound into coded signals representing frequency (or pitch), duration (or sound length), and intensity (or loudness) characteristics. Coded signals are transmitted via a *cable* to the transmission coil or headpiece. The *transmission coil* allows the internal and external components of the device to communicate by sending the coded signals as radio frequency waves across the scalp to the internal magnet of the receiver.

The *internal* part of the CI device—the portion your physician implanted during surgery—consists of a receiver-stimulator and an electrode array. The *receiver* collects the radio frequency waves from the headpiece and sends them to the stimulator. The *stimulator* converts the signal to electrical pulses before delivering the appropriate electrical energy to the electrode array inserted in the cochlea. The *electrode array* consists of a number of electrodes that wind through the cochlea, which is arranged like a piano keyboard going from high to low frequencies. Each electrode is associated with a range of frequencies. The electrode array stimulates the remaining auditory nerve fibers in the cochlea according to the characteristics of the coded signal. Electrical sound information is sent through the auditory system to the brain for interpretation.

Now you understand how the CI converts acoustic sound to an electrical signal that can be understood by the auditory system. However, each CI processes sound uniquely according to the user's listening limits and preferences. The next step is to determine what your child's listening limits are and how to help your child maximize his hearing abilities. This process begins at the initial stimulation appointment.

The audiologist will connect the external components and the internal components with the transmission coil during the initial stimulation appointment. Once your child is wearing the external equipment, the audiologist will connect the device to the computer via a cable and programming interface. This connection allows the audiologist to monitor both the internal and external parts of the CI system. Connection to the internal components allows your audiologist to determine how well electricity flows through the implanted portion of the device. Connection to the external components lets your audiologist set the program to which your child will listen.

Testing the Internal Component

Your audiologist will check the integrity of the internal device using *telemetry*, which assesses how well electricity flows at each electrode site in the electrode array. Your audiologist will determine and document which electrodes, if any, show open circuits (no flow of electricity), short circuits (too much flow of electricity), or high impedance (too little flow of electricity). Electrodes that do not let electricity flow properly will not be used in the MAP because they may distort the sound delivered by the CI. Such distortions will affect loudness growth, or how your child perceives sound as it changes from soft to comfortable to loud levels, which could affect his acquisition of speech awareness and recognition. Sometimes your audiologist may turn off an electrode when full insertion of the electrode array is not possible due to anatomical differences. The frequencies that would have been assigned to the electrodes that are turned off are then reallocated among the remaining electrodes. Because electrode impedance significantly impacts how your child perceives sounds through the CI and because it can change over time, impedance testing should be performed at each visit.

Programming the Speech Processor

Once the audiologist knows which electrodes to include in the MAP, programming of the speech processor can begin. The MAP should maximize how the CI changes acoustic sound into usable electricity for each electrode included in the MAP. The MAP settings are crucial to your child's ability to develop *speech perception*, the awareness and recognition of speech. The more closely the MAP represents sounds and speech, the better your child's chances of developing speech perception with the CI.

To create a MAP for your child's speech processor, your audiologist needs to find out the lowest and the most comfortable levels at which your child responds for each electrode. The least amount of electrical stimulation to which your child responds all of the time is called the *threshold level* (T-level). The amount of electrical stimulation that your child can listen to comfortably all of the time is called the *most comfortable level* (M-level). The amount of electrical stimulation that is loud but still comfortable is called the *comfortable level* (C-level). The difference between the softest sound to which your child responds (T-level) and the comfortable level of sound (C- or M-level) is called the *dynamic range*. The relationship among these levels of electrical stimulation is shown in Figure 7–1. All of these measures—threshold levels, comfort levels, and dynamic range—are crucial to matching the implant MAP to your child's responses to electrical stimulation, which will provide the best opportunity for your child to learn to understand speech.

Threshold (T-Level)

The threshold, or T-level, is the lowest level of electricity at each electrode that elicits an auditory response from your child. It is difficult for adults to acknowledge when they barely hear a sound, so imagine how much more difficult this task will be for your child! Some children who had residual hearing before getting the CI might immediately recognize sound, which happened with Caroline, a little girl whose hearing loss was identified shortly after birth and who received a CI before 3 years of age. Her mother recounts the initial stimulation appointment in *Journeys with Our Children* (The Moog Center for Deaf Education [Moog Center], 2006):

> Her implant was activated on October 6 and she was well on her way to hearing a new world of sounds from that day forward. It was such a fun and exciting day to watch Caroline's first reaction with a surprised look on her face and her little finger pointing at her ear when she first heard sound from the implant. (p. 43)

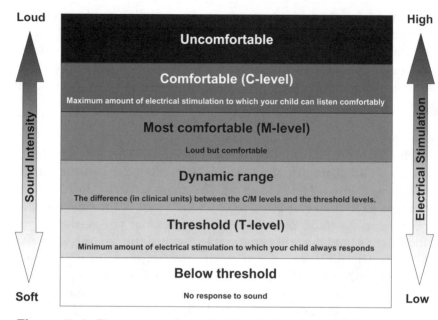

Loud ↑ Sound Intensity ↓ **Soft**

High ↑ Electrical Stimulation ↓ **Low**

Uncomfortable

Comfortable (C-level)
Maximum amount of electrical stimulation to which your child can listen comfortably

Most comfortable (M-level)
Loud but comfortable

Dynamic range
The difference (in clinical units) between the C/M levels and the threshold levels.

Threshold (T-level)
Minimum amount of electrical stimulation to which your child always responds

Below threshold
No response to sound

Figure 7–1. The range of comfort levels for your child's response to different levels of sound is shown. The light bands on the bottom of the figure represent sounds that your child cannot hear or that your child perceives as quiet or soft. The grey bands in the middle of the figure represent sounds that your child perceives as comfortable. The dark bands at the top of the figure represent sounds that your child perceives as too loud or uncomfortable. Sound intensity is shown on the left side of the figure. Electrical stimulation through the CI is shown on the right side of the figure. Scales for both sound intensity and electrical stimulation range from low levels at the bottom to high levels at the top. The parameters listed in the bands—threshold level, dynamic range, most comfortable, and comfortable levels—are used to set your child's CI program to maximize his ability to hear sounds and understand speech.

Not all children are able to respond so easily to sound. Right after implantation, young children often have trouble identifying the softest level at which they detect a sound. This is because they are unfamiliar with sound and have not developed sound awareness, the ability to tell whether a sound occurred or not. As a result, your child may not respond to very soft sounds during the initial stimulation appointment. Instead, she might wait for a louder sound requiring more electricity before she shows a reaction. Audiologists call this a *minimum response level* because it represents the softest intensity or lowest electrical stimulation level at which your child can *respond*. This is not necessarily the softest intensity of which he is *aware*. This is similar to the listening process of newborn babies with normal hearing. As your child matures and gains listening experience using the CI, his confidence with the decision of sound awareness will improve. As a result, your child's ability to detect very soft sounds that require lower energy levels will improve over time until your child can respond at his true threshold level.

Your audiologist understands that young children often provide a minimum response level rather than a true threshold. To account for this, your audiologist will set T-levels below where your child actually responds. The threshold-setting process is repeated for each electrode, one at a time. Your audiologist likely will start with an electrode that corresponds to a lower frequency signal, followed by one that matches with a higher frequency signal. This process will continue until your child no longer can provide reliable responses. If not all electrodes can be assessed, the computer software can estimate values of the untested electrodes to create the MAP. Threshold for remaining electrodes can be assessed during subsequent programming sessions (Figure 7–2).

Remember that as your child's ability to respond to very soft sounds changes over time, so will his threshold levels. Your child will acquire sound awareness by learning to listen. The best way that you can support your child's discovery of sounds and sound awareness is to provide a variety of listening experiences. This begins with your commitment to the listening process by having your child consistently wear the implant for 12 to 18 hours per day.

Comfortable Levels (C- and M-Levels)

Comfort levels include the electrical stimulation judged to be either most comfortable (M-level) or loud but comfortable (C-level) when the child listens to speech. Advanced Bionics and Med-El devices use the M-level for programming. Cochlear devices apply the C-level. Comfort levels are very important because they ensure that sounds do not get too loud for your child.

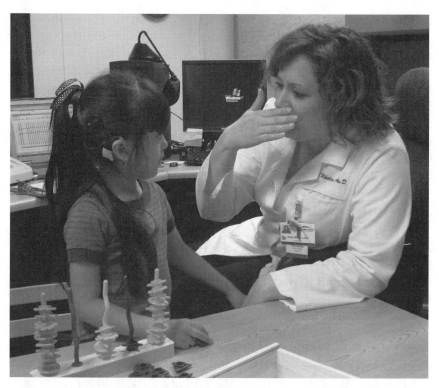

Figure 7–2. At a MAPping session, the audiologist wants to test how well Katherine hears. She hides her mouth so that Katherine doesn't get any visual cues and asks her to repeat what she says.

Very young children cannot tell the audiologist when a sound is comfortable, but they can indicate when a signal is too loud. They might not have the words to do this, but their reaction—a worried look, reaching for a parent, crying, startling, or removal of the magnet—speaks volumes. Your audiologist will be very careful to avoid presenting sounds that are too loud for your child for many reasons. Intense stimulation of an electrode could frighten your child, which could cause your child to distrust the audiologist and the device. A bad initial experience could negatively influence the rest of the initial stimulation appointment, participation in future programming appointments, and your child's future success using the implant. If high stimulation does happen, it is very important that you help your audiologist resume programming at lower levels to restore your child's trust with the audiologist and create a positive initial experience with the implant.

Just like threshold levels were set lower than the level at which your child responded, M- and C-levels will be set below the level at which the child responds negatively. After each electrode is set (or as many as can be accomplished during the appointment), all electrodes are tested at the comfort levels while your child sits and plays. Your child's behavior is observed and comfort levels are decreased if he seems uncomfortable. Just like with threshold levels, the best way for your child to learn which sounds are comfortable is by experiencing different sound levels. Your job is to expose him to a broad range of listening events.

Dynamic Range

The dynamic range includes sound intensity levels from threshold to the most comfortable level and represents the limits of sound that your child can hear comfortably. The dynamic range also lets your audiologist know how quickly sound grows from being very quiet to being too loud. The loudness of a sound should grow gradually, as it does for individuals with normal hearing. A small dynamic range means that loudness grows more quickly. This means your child may have trouble telling the difference between soft, comfortable, and loud sounds, which could limit your child's speech perception abilities. Your audiologist will probably set your child's dynamic range conservatively at first to make sure a loud sound does not frighten your child. As your child adjusts to listening with the device, your audiologist will steadily increase the dynamic range to allow the best opportunity for your child to develop speech perception.

Objective Measures

Sometimes, an infant or young child cannot (or will not) cooperate to let the audiologist know what he hears for one electrode, let alone all electrodes. This often happens with children who are too young to provide the information, who have no knowledge of sound, or who are unfamiliar with the programming process. If your child cannot reliably respond to sound or stimulation, your audiologist can use objective measures to make sure that the CI is providing the right amount of stimulation to your child's auditory system. Your child can even play or sleep when these measures are tested.

Each CI manufacturer uses its own technology to find out how the auditory nerve responds to stimulation by the electrode array. Cochlear Corporation uses Neural Response Telemetry (NRT); Advanced Bionics applies Neural Response Imaging (NRI); and Med-El utilizes Auditory Nerve Response Telemetry (ART). All three measures use radio-frequency waves to send a signal to the electrode array, which in turn stimulates the auditory nerve. The electrical activity generated by the auditory nerve is recorded by the electrodes and displayed on the computer monitor. Additionally, Electrical Stapedius Reflex Thresholds (ESRT) are used to approximate response levels. For ESRT, the stimulation level is increased until the stapedius muscle in the middle ear on the non-implant side contracts or tightens. This stapedial reflex occurs in both ears when a sound is loud but comfortable. You may need to help your child stay very still during the recording of the ESRT because movement, talking, or swallowing could disrupt the measurement. Luckily, all three measures can be collected quickly.

Objective measures like NRT, NRI, ART, and ESRT provide information about threshold and comfort levels, neural function, and device functionality. These measures are crucial when working with very young children who cannot provide reliable responses to sounds or stimulation. NRT, NRI, ART, and ESRT results generally agree with true threshold and comfort levels, but individual differences do exist. This is why it is so important that the audiologist gets your child's actual response to sound stimulation via threshold and comfort levels.

Creating the MAP

Once threshold and comfort levels have been established for a few electrodes, the computer will generate a MAP that details the electrical current levels for each electrode (Figure 7–3). This MAP, which is unique to your child's responses across the entire electrode array, is stored on a computer chip in the speech processor.

Once the MAP has been created, the microphone on the speech processor is activated so that your child will hear speech through the implant for the first time. This is the moment that you have envisioned since you made the decision toward cochlear implantation for

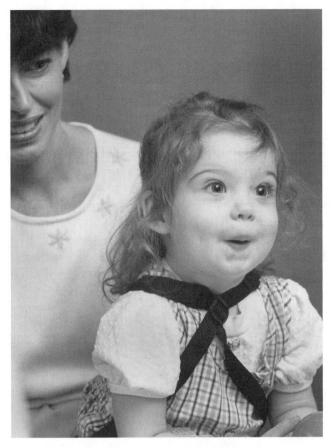

Figure 7–3. Emily is hearing sound for the first time at her initial stimulation session. Although she is delighted, not all children respond positively at first.

your child. Your child may meet your expectations by smiling and enjoying his early listening experience. On the other hand, your child might have little reaction to sound, as often is seen with very young CI recipients. The lack of a response does not mean the device is not working. Your child might have a negative reaction to the device. For example, your child might cry or try to remove the external device. A negative reaction does not mean that your child is in pain, nor does it indicate future use or benefit from the device. It most likely means that your child is surprised by or afraid of the new sounds he hears. Remember that suddenly hearing sound is a very different experience for your child, and it will take time to incorporate sound into his world. Try not to be disappointed or second guess your decision about implantation if your child's reaction does not meet your expectations. Instead, trust your audiologist and the CI team. Support your child by praising him for going through this process he likely does not understand.

Your audiologist will create new MAPs as your child gets (re)acquainted with sound and listening through the CI. All current CI devices can store more than one MAP on the speech processor. In the beginning, multiple MAPs allow the audiologist to provide progressively more stimulation with each MAP. This allows you to gradually increase the amount of electrical stimulation provided by the CI as your child adapts to wearing the device. One parent described how Eli, her 4-year-old child who wore a hearing aid in his left ear and received a CI in his right ear, reacted initially to the sound of the implant (Moog Center, 2006):

> Eli was excited about hearing with both ears again, but over the next few weeks and months, he really struggled. Everything was so loud to him in the implanted ear that he had to start each day with the smallest setting possible and let it build gradually. . . . Over time, his implant settings widened until, eventually, to our great delight, his right ear became his better ear. (p. 31)

Once your child has adjusted to using the CI, MAPs can be programmed for various listening situations—in quiet, in noise, or at school—by including different features in the MAP. Using multiple MAPs in this way will allow your child to maximize her ability to hear with the CI in different listening environments.

Subsequent Programming Appointments

Although the initial MAP settings are not ideal, they act as a starting point for future MAPs. Regular follow-up sessions allow the audiologist to adjust the MAP to your child's response to sound as she gets used to listening with the CI. Sounds that your child could not hear and sounds that were too loud during the initial stimulation may become comfortable as your child gains listening experience. Changes in stimulation levels happen relatively quickly in the beginning and will stabilize after your child's brain learns to use the electrical input.

Because changes occur quickly in the beginning, your audiologist will want frequent visits with your child to program the best MAP for your child. At each appointment, your audiologist will measure telemetry, threshold, and comfort levels to create two to four MAPs that match your child's listening needs. Your first two follow-up appointments will most likely occur weekly or monthly after initial stimulation of the device until an initial good MAP is set. Adjustments to your child's MAP will be scheduled at regular intervals, as shown in Table 7-1. These visit schedules are a rule of thumb, though, and your child may need more MAPping appointments as he learns how to listen.

Every child's pathway to responding to sound from the CI is different. In *Journeys with Our Children* (Moog Center, 2006), one parent recalls the story of her two children, Elena and Jacob, both of whom have received a CI (p. 60). Jacob progressively lost his hearing

Table 7–1. Frequency of cochlear implant MAPping appointments as a function of auditory experience with the cochlear implant

Months after Cochlear Implant Stimulation	Frequency of MAPping Appointments
0	Initial stimulation
0–1	Every 1–2 weeks
1–12	Every 1–3 months
12–36	Every 6 months
36+	Every 12 months

Note. The frequency of appointments for MAPping the speech processor decreases as your child gains listening experience with the CI. Months after CI stimulation are represented in the column on the left. Frequency of MAPping appointments is shown in the column on the right. The audiologist will see your child often during the first few months after the CI is activated to create a good initial MAP. MAPping sessions generally become less frequent over time, although additional appointments to fine-tune the speech processor can be scheduled as needed if your child's listening abilities or listening needs change.

before he was 1 year old and received his CI by age 2. He responded very well to new sounds:

> Jacob was fitted with a processor. The smile on his face brought tears to my eyes. He was able to hear again. He remembered many sounds that he had before he lost his hearing. Within two weeks, he was responding to sound very quickly and began progressing well in spoken language once again.

Elena, on the other hand, did not have the same experience. She was diagnosed with profound hearing loss soon after birth and received her CI at age 5 years. Her mother remembered that Elena hated the high frequencies but tolerated the low frequencies. "It took her over six months before she could be comfortable with high sounds and be able to use her processor more effectively" (p. 60).

Because each child learns to adapt to hearing new sounds differently, it is very important that you bring your child to follow-up visits and that you monitor your child's reaction to sounds and speech. Your daily interactions with your child will guide you. You may notice if your child stops responding to his name consistently. Your child might not respond to specific sounds, like an "s" or "sh" sound, suggesting that he needs more information in the high frequencies. Your audiologist needs to know how your child functions every day to adjust the stimulation levels of the MAP appropriately. Remember that your child will need time to adjust to any changes in the MAP. You can help by encouraging your child to try the new MAP even when she wants to revert to the old familiar settings. Explain that the only way to get used to the new MAP is to practice using the new settings, and praise your child for trying something new.

Test Procedures

Your audiologist will check the settings of your child's new MAP by testing her in a soundproof booth. One audiologist will present sound through the speakers and wait for a reaction from your child that will be confirmed by another audiologist inside the booth. For infants and very young children, the audiologist will watch your child's response to the presence and absence of sound. Your child may stop playing or eating, raise eyebrows, look up, glance toward you, or get a curious look on his face. The audiologist might teach your child to respond to sound by looking toward a toy that lights up, animates, or both. Older toddlers might be able to play with a toy in response to sound. For example, he might hold a block near his ear and toss it in a bucket as soon as she hears a sound. The type of testing depends on your child's age, auditory experience, and ability to cooperate with the task.

Most children show noticeable responses to speech during the initial stimulation appointment. These responses are based on sound awareness, or detection of the presence versus the absence of sound. It will take time and listening experience before your child can attach meaning to these sounds. Remember that the initial stimulation is the starting point of your child's journey in the hearing world. You may only see little changes at the start, but remember that from small beginnings come great things.

What to Expect from Your Child

Most young children who undergo cochlear implantation have little, if any, experience listening to sound. Because of your child's unfamiliarity with sound, he may not know how to react when sound is presented through the CI. Your child might have no reaction at all. He might show fear, alarm, confusion, or anxiety. Your child might cry from being overwhelmed. One parent described the response of Jake, her 14-month-old son, to sound in *Journeys with Our Children* (Moog Center, 2006): "His implant was activated a short time after the surgery and I remember him crying a little. It seemed to be some kind of reaction to sound. We were so thrilled about the possibility of him learning to speak and hear" (p. 13).

Others will exhibit a more positive response with happiness and excitement. An older child might widen his eyes with wonder at hearing sound (again), as happened with Eli, who lost his hearing at age 2 and received his implant almost 2½ years later:

> The day of his hook up, they took out his left hearing aid and started turning on the electrodes in his right ear while he played a game. But after a few minutes, Eli turned to us and said, "Would somebody please fix my hearing aid? It keeps beeping." We all laughed and told him, "That's not your aid; you're hearing through your implant." (Moog Center, p. 31)

The range of emotions and reactions from a child during the initial stimulation appointment depends on his age, hearing experience, and language development. It is difficult to predict exactly how your child will react, so you should be prepared for anything that might happen (Figure 7–4).

The audiologist will try to get your child to respond to sounds that are very soft (threshold level) and sounds that are comfortable (most comfortable or comfortable level) for several electrodes. Your child might not react purposely, but you might see eye widening; eyebrow raising; or cessation of sucking, eating, or playing. Your child might not be able to respond reliably to sound at all. Do not worry because the audiologist can use objective measures like NRT, NRI, ART, and ESRT to set the MAP for the CI, if needed.

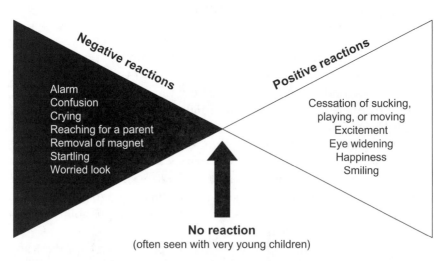

Figure 7–4. Children can respond a variety of ways to sound during the initial stimulation appointment. The black triangle on the left side of the figure represents negative reactions to sound through the CI. The intersecting point of the two triangles indicates no reaction to initial stimulation of the CI, a behavior more commonly seen in very young children. The white triangle on the right side of the figure characterizes positive responses to sound through the CI. A child's reaction to sound via initial stimulation of the CI depends on age, hearing experience, and language development.

The audiologist does not expect your child to use words in response to sound. Neither should you. As your child gains listening experience, she will become more confident and better able to respond reliably to sounds at soft and comfortable listening levels. The initial stimulation is the most challenging time to program the device because your child is unfamiliar with programming and with hearing in general. Just know that it will get easier over time.

Even if your child responds to electrical stimulation during the initial appointment, this does not mean your child can understand speech. Remember that your child has no reference point for sound. He needs to learn to listen, just like a newborn baby. Auditory skills build over time starting with sound awareness and ending with speech recognition. Sound *awareness* means that your child can tell whether a sound occurred or not. Your audiologist tests this by presenting sounds and speech and recording when your child responds to the signal. After your child can distinguish between presence and absence of sound, he can begin to work on sound discrimination. Sound *discrimination* refers to the ability to tell if two sounds are the same or different. Sound *identification*, the next step, means that your child can attach a label to the sound. The audiologist might ask your child to identify objects with names that differ in number of syllables (like ball, baby, and ice cream cone). This lets the audiologist know if your child can tell the difference between words based on syllable pattern. The final step of speech perception is for your child to achieve *comprehension*, or word understanding. This last step of the hierarchy is the goal you had in mind when you decided on cochlear implantation for your child. This is a long process that requires patience, persistence, and practice, but the rewards are great.

What to Expect from Yourself, the Parent

The otolaryngologist, audiologist, therapist, teacher, child, and parent all have roles that contribute to your child's success using the CI. The otolaryngologist surgically implants the device and assesses the medical aspects of the CI process. The audiologist manages your child's hearing abilities and her CI function and use. The speech-language pathologist monitors your child's speech, language, and communication skills. Each professional has a specific job and all work together to help your child function in the hearing world. Your main job as the parent of a child with a CI centers on your commitment to the entire process of cochlear implantation.

Monitor Your Child's Communication Abilities

Your commitment to the CI process begins with your child. You are responsible for monitoring your child's performance every time she tries a new MAP. Your child's auditory or speech skills may improve, decrease, or not change at all in response to a program change. Note any changes that immediately follow use of a new MAP. It might help to keep a diary of your child's reactions to sound. Report these changes to the audiologist, who can incorporate your feedback into subsequent programming sessions.

Attend All Follow-Up Appointments

The best way for your child to adapt to listening with the CI is for her to wear the device during all waking hours. As your child gains listening experience, the brain adapts to the signal provided by the CI. This causes his listening needs to change. These changes will occur more frequently during the first year after implantations. To accommodate the brain's adaptation to sound and to expand your child's dynamic range (remember, a broader dynamic range is associated with better speech understanding), your audiologist needs to adjust the MAP on the speech processor. You should pledge to your child that you will bring her to the follow-up appointments with the audiologist, speech-language pathologist, otolaryngologist, and other professionals to provide the best opportunity for your child to develop communication skills similar to those of hearing children.

Monitor Your Child's Physical Well-Being

Especially right after the initial stimulation appointment, you will need to check the skin under the magnet daily. Some parents worry that the magnet will fall off, so they tighten the magnet too much.

This could cause the skin under the magnet to die, a condition called *necrosis*, which you want to avoid. Only your audiologist should change the magnet strength. Remember that the transmission coil might fall off during the first few days. The more your child wears the device, the greater the magnet attraction between the transmission coil and the internal receiver. Be aware that because this is a magnet; it will be attracted to other magnetic sources like wheelchairs and some highchairs. You and your child will learn to replace the transmission coil should it fall off. Pay attention if the transmission coil repeatedly falls off, but try not to overtighten the magnet because it could have a negative effect on the underlying skin.

Manage Your Child's Equipment

You will receive information about how the CI device works and how to assess its function. You need to know how to turn on the device, switch programs, and change the volume. It is very important that you know how to troubleshoot the device by checking the battery, microphone, transmission coil, and other parts. You should also maintain a supply of parts such as batteries, cables, a headset, and backup processor for your child. You want to have these parts on hand in case of equipment difficulties to avoid your child being "off the air."

Inform Your Child's Teacher/Caregiver

Teachers and caregivers who are in direct contact with your child should also have some knowledge of the care and maintenance of your child's CI. Because batteries, cables, and the transmission coil can become weak or break down at school or daycare, make sure that the facility has a supply of parts as well.

Cover Your Child's Equipment

Your child's CI standardly comes with a 3-year manufacturer's warranty that includes repairs and one loss of the device. You need to know when this service contract expires so you can arrange for coverage of your child's CI device through a manufacturer or other company. Make sure that you are clear on which device parts are covered under the warranty and if this includes repairs, loss, or accidental damage.

Keep the Focus on Your Child

Your commitment to the CI process not only begins with your child, but also ends with your child. Make sure that the initial stimulation appointment and follow-up appointments are all about your child. This is a special time for both of you. Let your child know that you are dedicated to helping her hear to the best of his ability. Once your child sees your devotion to the CI process, he will follow your lead.

The initial stimulation is a much anticipated appointment because it is the first time your child will be exposed to sound. Be realistic about what to expect from your child during this session. Remember, the initial stimulation is merely the first step in your child's long journey toward independent communication. You have chosen cochlear implantation for your child. To achieve the end result of independent communication, you must support your child's lifelong endeavor by attending appointments, ensuring functioning equipment, and monitoring your child's performance. Your commitment as a family to the process is key to your child's progress with the CI. As Harry Emerson Fosdick said, "He who chooses the beginning of the road chooses the place it leads to. It is the means that determines the end."

References

Berke, J. (2007, December 17). *Cochlear implant hookup experience.* Retrieved March 6, 2008, from http://www.deafness.about.com/od/basics ofcochlearimplants/a/cihookup.htm

Boys Town National Research Hospital. (2008). Pediatric cochlear implant program—Initial stimulation. Retrieved March 6, 2008, from http://www. boystownhospital.org/Cochlear/Pediatric/initial.asp

Firszt, J. B., & Reeder, R. M. (1996). Cochlear implants and children: Device programming and considerations for young children. *Seminars in Hearing, 17*(4), 337–351.

Gordon, K., Papsin, B. C., & Harrison, R. V. (2004). Programming cochlear implant stimulation levels in infants and children with a combination of objective measures. *International Journal of Audiology,43*(Suppl. 1), S28-S32.

The Moog Center for Deaf Education. (2006). *Journeys with our children.* St. Louis, MO: Author.

Moore, J. A., & Teagle, H. F. B. (2002). An introduction to cochlear implant technology, activation, and programming. *Language, Speech, and Hearing Services in Schools, 33*(3), 153-161.

Plapinger, D. (2006). A broader view of cochlear implants. *The ASHA Leader, 11*(8), 5-13.

Tharpe, A. M., & Sladen, D. (2004). How we do it: Keeping paediatric patients motivated during the cochlear implant rehabilitative process. *Cochlear Implants International, 5*(1), 2-8.

Chapter 8

Auditory-Verbal Communication: Why We Recommend It

By Melissa H. Sweeney

The parent of a child who is deaf once said, "Life is meant to be lived out loud." That statement, of course, has significant meaning for children who are deaf and wear cochlear implants.

Factors That Affect Children's Progress

When parents investigate the option of a cochlear implant (CI) for their child, they hope that this device will have a positive impact on communication skills. They often ask, "Will my child talk?" and "When will my child talk?"

Overall, children who receive CIs will demonstrate various levels of benefit. It is important for you to have appropriate and high, but realistic, expectations for your child. Several factors are known to influence how children will benefit from a CI and what kind of progress can be expected. Some of these factors are:

- Age at implantation
- Duration of hearing loss
- Cognitive skills

- Normal inner ear
- Child's mode of communication (speech, signing, or both)
- Communication method at school and at home
- Additional diagnoses or disorders that affect a child's ability to learn or develop speech and the functional use of residual hearing
- Language and communication abilities
- The family's commitment to and involvement in the rehabilitative process.

Research has demonstrated that a younger age at implantation allows for better speech perception and spoken language skills (Colletti et al., 2005; Dettman, Pinder, Briggs, Dowell, & Leigh, 2007; Kirk et al., 2002; Robbins, Koch, Osberger, Zimmerman-Phillips, & Rabin, 2004). The brain is most "plastic," or accepting of new information, when a child is young (about 3 years old). Children who receive CIs before the age of 3 usually demonstrate "normal central auditory maturation" within 6 months of implant use. A normal auditory pathway is likely to be necessary for the development of speech and language skills (Sharma et al., 2005).

How long a child has had a hearing loss often mirrors age at implantation for children: the shorter the length of time our brains have been unstimulated by sound, the better.

If a child has additional diagnoses or disorders that affect her learning abilities or communication development, her progress with a CI or level of benefit is expected to be affected, because using a CI is a learning process (Holt & Kirk, 2005). In other words, children who have any diagnosis that indicates that they learn at a slower rate can be expected to progress at a slower rate in the development of their listening, language, and speech skills.

A child's communication skills at the time of implantation are also an important factor. Young children are expected to demonstrate certain nonverbal communication skills (engaging in eye contact, turn taking), even if they do not possess a formal language system (formal sign language or spoken words). Of course, the older the child, the more important the formal language system is. Oral motor skills are also considered in prognoses for children receiving CIs. Difficulty with oral motor skills, that is, moving the lips, teeth, or tongue appropriately, will influence a child's speech production.

Research has shown that children who are in environments where speech is used and that focus on listening have better speech perception and spoken language outcomes overall (Tobey, Rekart, Buckley, & Geers, 2004). This does not mean that every child with a CI should be in educational environments that do not use any visual language (sign language). Many factors should be considered when determining educational placement for children with CIs, including the skills they possess and their need for auditory experiences.

From experience, our program has seen the importance of family participation in the rehabilitative process, and it cannot be emphasized enough how crucial family participation is. The better educated and informed you are, and the more active you are in your child's rehabilitation process, the more successful your child will be. Consistent use during all waking hours, except in water, of an appropriately MAPped CI speech processor is also essential for a child to benefit from the CI. Regular check-ups with your child's audiologist, during which you provide information about your child's responses to sounds and progress, will ensure this (Figure 8–1).

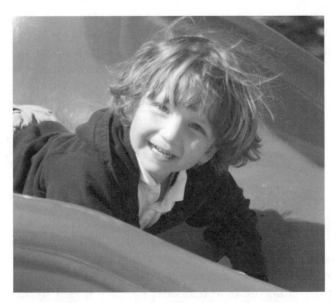

Figure 8–1. Ben is an active boy who participates in many playground activities, like the slide.

Why Is an Auditory Based-Rehab Program Important?

When you are trying to make decisions about communication options and educational placements for your child, it is important to be well informed about all of your options. First, identify your communication and educational goals for your child. It is easier to make a plan when you know where you want to go. Do you want your child to attend a mainstream school program? Do you want your child to become a proficient spoken language communicator, or is your goal for your child to develop some speech to use in addition to sign language, which is her main means of communication? These are important questions to ask, but remember, your answers must be realistic. Your CI professionals can help you work through these questions and develop realistic answers.

Several communication options exist for children with hearing loss. American Sign Language (ASL) is a visually-based language. Speech and hearing are not used. Spoken English and ASL cannot be used simultaneously because ASL has its own word order and grammar. Exclusive use of ASL is not conducive to CI use. Total Communication (TC) is a communication system using signed language with speech. TC programs vary as to the emphasis that is placed on visual information (signing) and speech. In other words, some TC programs may use more speech than others. Remember, CI users require speech and listening to be emphasized in order for them to receive the maximum benefit from their device. Cued speech is a system that uses hand shapes representing speech sounds in combination with speech. Auditory oral communication emphasizes the use of listening with verbal communication, along with speech reading and lip reading. Auditory-Verbal Communication is an option for families of children who are deaf or hard of hearing to develop spoken language through listening alone, without the use of formal visual communication (sign language or speech reading). Auditory-Verbal practice has guiding principles that include early identification of hearing loss and aggressive management of hearing loss, including the use of state-of-the art technology. Families are encouraged and guided by the professional to help their child use hearing as the primary means for developing spoken language without the use of formal visual communication (sign language or speech reading). Parents become the child's primary teachers of listening and spoken language. Consistent participation of the family in individualized therapy sessions is essential to help families create listening environments that allow their child to integrate listening and spoken language into all aspects of life. Auditory-Verbal therapy emphasizes the natural development of listening, language, cognition, and communication. Families learn to help their child self-monitor spoken language through listening. Ongoing formal and informal diagnostic assessments are used by the therapist to provide feedback to the family and to monitor the child's progress. Auditory-Verbal therapists promote education in regular classrooms with typical hearing peers using appropriate support services (Estabrooks, 2006).

There is not one single approach that is right for every child with a CI. Making the decision as to which approach is right for your child must be based on your goals for your child, the factors that influence your child's use of a CI, and what is realistic for your child. All of these considerations should be discussed with the professionals working with your child. You can find more information about communication approaches in *Choices in Deafness* (Schwartz, 2007).

Based on our experiences and the existing research, our program recommends a rehabilitation program that is based on hearing. Children with CIs require intensive listening practice to develop good, functional auditory skills. For children who are appropriate, the Auditory-Verbal approach is ideal. Some children and families may not be appropriate for a pure Auditory-Verbal approach, for a variety of reasons. However, the general principles of Auditory-Verbal approach and the common strategies used are beneficial to all children who receive CIs.

Where Do We Start?

After your child's CI is stimulated (turned on), she will be receiving new auditory information that she may or may not recognize as sound. Remember, responding to sounds and recognizing sounds are learned skills that must be practiced. This ability does not develop automatically for children who receive CIs. A focus on auditory skill development is necessary. The ultimate goal of auditory rehabilitation is to teach your child to listen with her CI and to utilize these listening skills in every environment, not just the therapy room. Listening with the CI is a learning process.

To start this process of learning to listen with a CI, your child must wear the device during all waking hours from the very beginning, except when she is bathing or swimming. It is critical that the child wear the device consistently in order for the auditory pathway to develop and for the child's brain to receive this auditory stimulation and become accustomed to this information. Brains that have not been stimulated do not understand this auditory information because they have not had the "practice" that the CI is providing. Brains inexperienced with sound can forget this information, what it means, and how to use it easily. In other words, if the device is not worn consistently, it is hard for the brain to start building memory for these sounds.

Development of Listening Skills

How does listening develop? Erber (1982) described a listening continuum of "detection, discrimination, identification and comprehension." These skills are overlapping and build on each other. Detection means being aware of sound. Discrimination is the ability to recognize that there is a difference between sounds. Identification is recognizing a specific sound. Comprehension is understanding the sound and using it meaningfully. Since Erber's description of listening skills development, many other versions have followed that are based on his principles but may use other words to describe the concepts. See the list of resources for more information.

Detection

Detection is the first and essential skill a child must learn in order to progress. How does one teach a child to detect a sound? Initially, point out sounds to your child and draw her attention to sounds as they occur. For example, when the phone rings, try to get your child's attention, point to your ear, say "I hear that," and, as the phone continues to ring, take your child to show her what the sound is and name the object ("I hear the telephone"). Note what you just did. First, you emphasized the act of *listening* to the sound before you pointed to the object that produced it. This is a very important habit for you, the caregiver, to develop. The auditory information must be emphasized and focused on first before identifying the source of the sound. Emphasizing listening highlights the importance of sound and requires the child to begin to use listening to gain information. It is also a good strategy if you imitate the sound ("Sshhhhhh" whispered when you turn on the faucet and the water is running). Our goal is to teach your child to listen with a CI, so listening is always first and is the main focus.

How do you know if a child is really hearing the sounds? It is important to watch your child's behavior(s) when the sound is occurring. Parents and caregivers know their child's typical behaviors and responses. When the sound occurs, does your child's behavior change? The behavior may not be an obvious turn of the head, but something more subtle, such as eye shifting, sucking on pacifier/bottle, stopping the sucking on pacifier or bottle, quieting if she is vocalizing, or vocalizing if she is quiet. Pediatric audiologists and speech pathologists with experience working with children who have CIs are experts in identifying these behaviors, and parents will become experts too by paying close attention to the child's responses. But remember, initially, the child's behavior may not change in response to sounds, because listening and responding to sound is a learned skill. So, when you don't see the response you were hoping for, go back to getting the child's attention, pointing to your ear, and showing the child the source of the sound.

In the beginning, you will want to point out all sounds that occur around you: people talking, water running, the doorbell ringing, or someone hammering outside your house. Teach your child that these sounds are interesting and fun! Do not be discouraged if your child does not seem to be responding to sounds at first. Remember, listening and responding takes practice. The information your child is hearing with the CI is new and different. Over time, you will want to see if your child responds to these sounds by herself without you pointing them out. But remember this will take a little time.

A conditioned play response is another important skill to teach your child. Children who are 2 years of age and older can learn this skill. But again it takes practice (some children can learn this skill as early as 18 months of age). A conditioned play response is simply teaching your child to respond to a sound in a predetermined way. You may have seen your audiologist use this in testing your child. Games that you can use for this type of activity include something as simple as putting a block in a bucket or bowl, putting a puzzle piece in the puzzle, nesting toys, or shooting baskets with a basketball and hoop. The activity used has to be something that the child can do quickly and easily but is still fun. First, seat your child at a table or in a high chair and sit beside him on the side of his CI. Give him the piece or toy that you are going to use and have him put it to his ear, like he is listening and waiting for a sound (Figure 8-2). Do not let him perform the task until the sound has occurred. To teach this task, there must be a third person present to help train the child. The model (the person demonstrating the response for the child) and the person making the sound cannot be the same person; otherwise, the child will interpret this as "When I make a sound, I put the block in the bucket" and not "When I hear the sound, I put the block in the bucket." You will want the model to hold a toy as well and put it by his ear, so the child sees what he is to do. Then *make sure the child is unable to see the person who will produce the sound* and produce the sound. When the sound is provided, the model should put the block in the bucket (or whatever the activity you selected) and point to his ear saying, "I heard that." Hopefully, the child will do the same. Repeat

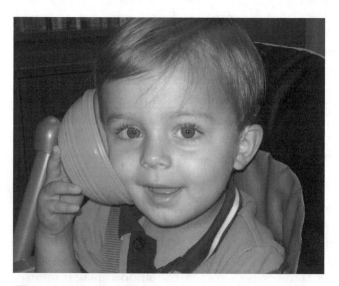

Figure 8–2. A simple listening activity: Charlie holds a plastic toy up to his ear and listens for a sound. When he hears a sound, he puts the toy on the table.

this to give the child another chance to practice, and then try to do this without a model, so that the child has to do it by himself. If the child is successful, congratulations; you have just taught your child his first important listening skill! If the child does not seem to respond quickly, you can try again with the model. Remember, it takes practice. You may be wondering, what sounds do I use? Use the Ling Six Sounds ("ah," "ee," "oo," "sh," "ss," and "mm") (Ling, 1989). These sounds are used because they will help you to make sure your child is hearing across the speech spectrum (low pitched sounds to high pitched sounds). You do not want to raise your voice when producing these sounds, but produce them at a normal conversational level.

What if my child is not 2 years of age or is not able to do this kind of activity? Using these same Ling Six Sounds ("ah," "ee," "oo," "sh," "ss," and "mm"), you can see if your child looks for these sounds when you make them during a play activity. Again, make sure that your child is not able to see you. Try positioning your child in a high chair or another chair and stand behind her and make the sound. When the child appears as if she is hearing the sound, then play and interact with your child to reward her for her listening.

Checking your child's responses to the Ling Six Sounds should be done every day. This is a quick, useful listening check for detection. Keep track of the responses you observe in your child. Maybe your child responds to a couple of the sounds at first but then begins to respond to other sounds. Because you know your child's typical responses to sounds, this will help you provide information to the professionals working with your child. What if the child doesn't appear to respond? Make sure your child was paying attention and not just distracted. This is possible when a child is very young or a new listener. If you feel the child is paying attention but not responding as she typically does, the implant may not be working. Try some of the troubleshooting strategies that your implant center has shown you and look in your guides from the manufacturer or on their Web sites. Once you have done this, then try the listening check again and see if the responses are different. If you still have concerns, contact your child's CI center. Eventually, raise your expectation for your child to imitate the sounds. If your child wears bilateral CIs, you should perform a listening check with your child wearing each speech processor independently.

Keep a notebook! Make notes on all of the sounds that you observe your child responding to (or detecting) and the way you noticed that she responded. It is also helpful to note, on a daily basis, sounds that she appears not to respond to. Make notes if she responded without you drawing her attention to the sound first, or if she required you to get her attention first. You will also want to keep track of whether your child not only looks for the sound but also recognizes it. See the identification section at the end of this chapter for more. The notebook is a great way to monitor progress over time, and this gives you good information to report to your audiologist and the speech pathologist.

Remember, detection (or responding to the sound, not recognizing what it is) is your child's first step. She must detect it before she can identify what it is.

Discrimination

Discrimination is perceiving differences in sounds. It is important for you to note if your child responds differently to different sounds. Specific skills in discrimination are typically addressed when it appears a child is having difficulty recognizing that there is a difference between sounds or words that are very similar (*apple* versus *apples*).

Identification

Identification is recognizing a sound, possibly by pointing to a picture, selecting a toy, or imitating the sound. There is a "hierarchy of acoustic contrasts" (Sindrey, 1997) that children systematically progress through as they develop identification skills (information adapted from Sindrey, 1997; Estabrooks, 2000; & Erber 1982):

- Differing suprasegmentals (duration, rate, pitch, intensity, stress)
  - Example: "Up up up" (said with rising pitch) versus "Weeeeeee" (said with falling pitch)
- Words differing in number of syllables
  - Example: *cup* versus *birthday cake*
- Words with the same syllable number, but differing consonant and vowel information
  - Example: *shoe* versus *ball*

■ Words with the same initial consonant sounds, but differing vowel sounds
  ■ Example: *ball* versus *bowl*
■ Words that have initial consonant sounds differing by manner
  ■ Example: *wall* versus *ball*
■ Words that have final consonants differing by manner
  ■ Example: *bone* versus *boat*
■ Words that have final consonants differing by voicing
  ■ Example: *back* versus *bag*
■ Words that have initial consonants differing by voicing
  ■ Example: *pea* versus *bee*
■ Words that have initial consonants differing by place
  ■ Example: *pool* versus *cool*
■ Words that have final consonants differing by place
  ■ Example: *knife* versus *nice*

Begin with the suprasegmental aspects of sounds. Suprasegmentals include pitch (high, medium, or low pitch), intensity (loud or quiet), or duration (long or short sounds, one syllable versus three syllables). Sounds that vary significantly in their suprasegmental aspects ("up up up" [three short, fast sounds, with a rising pitch] versus "wheeee" [one long sound with falling pitch]) are easiest to distinguish between or identify. In other words, your child will imitate the pitch and patterns of your speech before she is able to imitate the specific speech sounds you use. Hearing babies are able to imitate the suprasegmental aspects of speech sounds as young as 6 months of age. Using sounds that contrast in these ways during play will ultimately help facilitate your child's understanding.

The segmental aspects of speech include manner cues, that is, the way the speech sound is made, for example, stopping the airflow in "buh" or a continuous airflow in "ss," voicing cues (if the vocal cords are vibrating ["duh"] or not ["tuh"]), and place cues (where the speech sound is made on the lips or in the back of your throat) of speech sounds. Skill in identifying sounds can be improved using "Learning to Listen Sounds" (Estabrooks, 2006). Learning to Listen Sounds are onomatopoeias, or sounds that are words like *quack*. These sounds can be used to facilitate understanding of speech sounds, as well as for practicing the production of different speech sounds. Other examples of Learning to Listen Sounds are *moo* for the cow or *beep beep* for the car. You can find more information about Learning to Listen Sounds in resources by Estabrooks and other Auditory-Verbal therapy books. Use these sounds during play repeatedly to give the child plenty of opportunities to hear the sounds over and over and begin to remember and learn what sounds are associated with the objects and toys (Figure 8–3). During these activities, you will also want to encourage more imitation from your child. Remember, present the sound (say "moo") before you show what object goes with the sound. And this is also a great opportunity to provide other language for the child to listen to. For example, say "moo" without the child seeing your face or lips or the cow and pause. Look for the child's response. You can point to your ear and say "I heard a cow; it said 'mooooo.'" Again, note how your child is responding. You can ask your child, "Did you hear the cow say 'mooooo'?" and then bring the toy cow out and

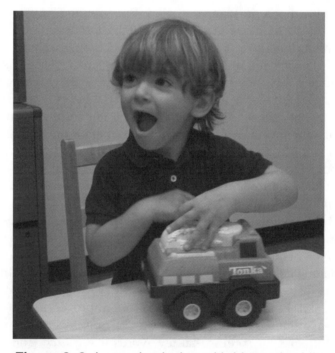

Figure 8–3. Logan is playing with his truck while the auditory-verbal therapist is talking. Logan demonstrates he is listening by making a big O sound.

repeat "mooo" and give it to the child to play with. As the child is play-ing, you can narrate in short phrases and sentences what he is doing. Remember to pause and give him an opportunity to take a turn. Use some other Learning to Listen Sounds, such as lip smacking as you make the toy cow eat, or "sshhhhh" as you make the toy cow sleep, and continue narrating what you are doing with the child ("The cow is sleeping. Sshhh.").

To check your child's identification of some of these Learning to Listen Sounds, a clean-up activity is a great, natural way to do this. Ini-tially, put two to three toys or other objects in front of the child and ask her to "clean up the cow," for example, and have a box for her to put the object in as she successfully cleans up. Make sure you allow your child to be successful at selecting the correct item, especially at the beginning. If she selects the wrong item, then you can cue the child to get the correct one by not taking the object from her or not allowing her to actually put it in the box. Repeat your direction and point to the correct toy or object when necessary. Then repeat the name of the object you have just talked about ("Bye-bye, cow").

After your child has demonstrated an understanding of some of these sounds, see if she can identify important people when they are named ("Mama"), identify important objects ("bottle"), and iden-tify significant words ("bye-bye"). The next step would be for the child to recognize two important words in a phrase ("mama's purse," "daddy's shoe").

Make note of the speech sounds your child is able to imitate (when she is not able to see your face). For example, if your child always produces "buh" for "puh," make note of it. Imitation is an important aspect of your child's listening development. Practicing saying what one hears and monitoring that the production matches what was said is a very important skill for the child to have.

How can I help my child improve imitation of speech sounds? Whisper voiceless speech sounds, for example, /p, t, h, s, k/ or the Learning to Listen Sounds made up of voiceless consonants such as in *pop* or *hop*. Whispering the voiceless sounds emphasizes that aspect of the sound. Repeat the sound that the child imitated incorrectly. For example, if the child says "dig" for "*big*," you could say "It's *b—b-b- big*. It's *big*." You have repeated the sound the child had trouble with and then also repeated the word in its natural context so that the child hears that as well. You must also take into account your child's age when looking at her imitation skills. Certain speech sounds develop later than others and this must be considered to have appropriate expectations. Talk with your speech-language professional about speech production order or see *Speech and the Hearing Impaired Child* (Ling, 2002).

Comprehension

Comprehension is your child's ability to understand and use the information she hears. For example, is your child able to understand common phrases ("It's all gone" or "Let's go bye-bye")? Then establish if your child is able to follow simple directions ("Go get your shoes") and then two-step directions ("Get the ball and throw it to me"). Is your child able to understand a variety of labels (people, foods, toys, clothing), action words (*walk, run, eat*), descriptors (*big, hot, yellow*), and location words (*in, under, over*)? Can she understand these words when they are combined in phrases ("a big yellow ball")? Can your child, answer *what, who,* and *where* questions? Continue to monitor your child's language development with your speech-language pathologist. Make note of the sentences your child utters. Remember to keep adding this information to your notebook.

Strategies and Activity Ideas

Strategies

There are many strategies you can use with your child to help her begin on her listening journey. No matter what the activity, the following strategies will help you to teach your child listening and spoken language skills:

1. Child wears device during all waking hours
2. Perform daily listening checks
3. Be aware of your environment for listening and communication opportunities
4. Use repetition
5. Emphasize listening and use hearing as the primary means of giving information to your child

6. Play
7. Use dialogue
8. Comment, rather than question; expand and pause
9. Provide your child natural opportunities to communicate
10. Observe and take note of the child's responses to sounds
11. Remember the listening levels and acoustic contrasts

Most importantly, make sure your child is always wearing the CI (except in the water). Check equipment regularly, keep extra batteries with you, follow the manufacturer's recommendations, and listen to the microphone to ensure the child is listening to the best possible sound at all times. Perform a listening check daily using the Ling Six Sounds.

Be aware of the sounds and noises in the environment when you are communicating or working with your child. Remember, it is easier to listen and to learn to listen in a quieter environment than in a noisy one. A new listener will not be able to identify which sound is the important sound (or which sound to focus on) if the environment has too many competing sounds and there is too much background noise. Make sure you are using a voice that has melody and is pleasant for a child to listen to. Repetition is essential for children to learn and understand the new information their CI is providing them. There is no need to raise your voice for a child with a CI or unnaturally emphasize words. It is more beneficial for a child to listen to naturally produced words and sentences.

Repetition is something that children need to learn language. Common phrases and words used throughout each day are important tools for teaching language. *Hot, push, open, eat, more,* and *up* are a few common words that can be used with children throughout the day during many different activities. Think of all the ways you can use the word *open.* You open the door of the car, you open the door on the refrigerator, you open the door of the dryer, you open the toy box, and you open the box of cereal. Repeating words and saying things the same way in the beginning of this journey will help your child develop a memory for words and understand what they mean.

Always focus on auditory information first. Remember, before you show your child what is making the sound, make sure she is listening to it. For example, if you are playing with Learning to Listen Sounds, hide the toy in your hands and make the sound a few times before you show her that toy. Giving her the toy to play with is the "reward" for participating and listening in that activity (Figure 8–4).

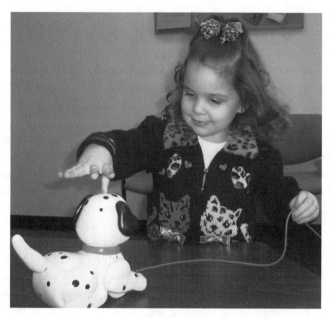

Figure 8–4. Emma is learning words while playing with a toy dog in auditory-verbal therapy.

Point to your ear and say "Listen, I hear that." If you find that you are showing your child what it is you were talking about, remember to say the phrase or sentence again to allow her that listening practice.

Play is very important with all children. This is how a child learns! A common question is "What kind of toys should I buy for my child?" The type of toy is not as important as how it is played with. The quality of the play is more important than the toy you use. If you follow the interests of the child, the child will be more engaged in the activity and more likely to listen, participate, and learn. With time, you will become better and better at incorporating these strategies into play with your child.

Use a dialogue when communicating and playing with your child. This means you and your child take turns making eye contact, vocalizing, and pointing to pictures. Obviously, you may initially feel like you are doing most of the talking, but that is okay. Comment about what your child is doing or looking at. Do not ask questions repeatedly. Asking questions puts the child in a test situation ("What's that?" "What's this?"). Commenting allows you, as the language model, to provide input for the child. Children need a lot of input, especially in the beginning. Pause after you say something, wait for a "response" from your child, which may be eye contact or a vocalization, and then take your next turn, which will be something verbal, just as you do in other conversations. Games that facilitate turn-taking are games like patty cake, peek-a-boo, rolling a ball back and forth, pushing a car back and forth, or book reading.

Provide rich language environments for your child throughout each day. Model language at, and slightly above, your child's language level. Use repetition, expanding (adding a little more information to your child's utterance), and rephrasing of the child's utterance (providing new information). Comment about what the child is doing or how the toy looks. Do not use test type questions ("What's that?") over and over. If your child points to a picture and says "car," reply by saying something such as "Yes, it's a big car." Use the Learning to Listen Sounds and talk about the toy, but do not question the child. Use speech that is pleasant to listen to, a rate of speech that is not fast and not slow, and speak at a normal conversational level. For example, if you have chosen to play with farm animals, before showing the child the toy as you bring it out of the box or the barn, say "Moo" and pause if the child is a brand new listener. Then, point to your ear again and say "Moo, I hear a cow" before you bring the cow out of the box. Say "Hi, cow" and wave to the cow.

Repeat "moo." Then present the cow to the child and see how she responds. Maybe the child says "moo" or something close to "moo." If not, you can repeat "The cow says 'moo.'" Then talk in simple ways about the cow, his color, his size, and what he's doing.

Make sure you are creating situations in which your child has a real reason to talk and communicate with you. When your child drops something, rather than picking it up automatically, allow the child the opportunity to tell you that she needs it. Maintain an expectation that your child will respond to sounds and that she will communicate with you. Of course, the level at which the child is able to communicate will change over time, so keep raising your expectations as your child's communication skills improve. The child's attempt may initially be a vocalization just to get your attention, but then become the use of a word such as "Mama" or "help" or "please," and then the use of two words together.

Activities

Some of the favorite activities that have been used in our clinic programs over time have been natural, play activities that are enjoyable for the child as well as the caregiver. One favorite is book reading. Book reading is ideal because you can position yourself in a natural way where the child is not able to see your face and has to rely on listening. Let the child sit in your lap and place the book in the child's lap so that you are both able to see the pages. Now you are positioned close to the child's ear and ready for a great listening and language activity. Use the same strategies that have been discussed already, such as commenting, pausing, and expanding. Remember the acoustic contrasts to help you effectively emphasize specific aspects of speech that may be necessary for your child. Lift-the-flap books are always fun and already have a built-in way to hide what you are talking about. Children's books often have good rhythm and melody that children enjoy listening to, and they often contain repetitive language for the child to hear multiple times. Often, you will encounter new vocabulary that you wouldn't otherwise have used had you not been reading this interesting book with your child.

Another favorite activity is singing and music (Figure 8–5). Parents often ask if their child will enjoy music or participate in musical activities. Music is a wonderful activity for children with CIs for many reasons. Singing encourages good breath control for speech, which encourages good vocal quality. It also varies suprasegmental aspects such as long and short durations, pitch variations, and intensity variations. Many children's songs also help to develop auditory memory because of the repetition. Many songs repeat lines and phrases, which the child is able to learn. Initially, it is a good idea to sing songs that use movements with them, such as "Itsy Bitsy Spider." See if the child attempts the movements or attempts to vocalize with the songs. Repetition of these songs will allow the child to learn them. Another idea to try is to start singing the song (after you feel like the child has heard it and is able to recognize it) without the movements. Observe if the child starts to perform the motions (then you join in), and this will tell you the child recognizes the song even before he can verbally name the song.

Cooking is another favorite. Making cookies is a fun example. You can start by announcing, "Let's make cookies," and observe your child's response. You could vary the vocabulary if your child is beyond this

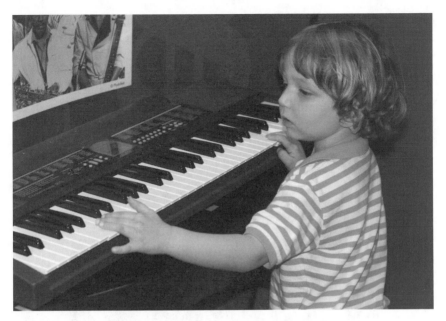

Figure 8–5. Ben loves to play the piano.

stage by saying, "Let's bake cookies." Then open the refrigerator door
and say "It's cold, brrrrr," remembering to give the child an opportunity to take a conversational turn (maybe she will laugh, so you repeat
it, and pause again, or maybe the child will imitate you or produce her
own verbalization, and then respond to her). Get the cookie dough
out of the refrigerator and open it and talk about how to open it. Do
you need a knife, can you "puuuullll" it open, or is it covered in a
bowl? You will also want to add a few "What should we do next?"
questions in your activity, and then pause, of course, to give the child
an opportunity to respond. If the child does not respond, you fill in
the "answer" ("I know, let's roooooll it"). As you roll out the cookie
dough with a rolling pin say "Roll, roll, roll," and then cut out some
cookies with cookie cutters. Say "push" (whispered) to emphasize the
voiceless aspects of the speech sounds. Then, put the cookies "on"
the cookie sheet and put them in the oven that is "hot, hot, hot" while
blowing on your finger. Set the timer, of course, and then listen for the
timer so you know the cookies are ready. Blow on the cookies to cool
them off and remove them from the tray. You can frost them with
icing using different colors. Can your child label the colors, can she

repeat the vowel sounds in the words? Remember what is appropriate for your child's level. Then use a dull knife to spread on the icing. Cooking is a great way to target any language concept or listening skill (Figure 8-6).

Art activities are also great. You can use a glue stick and go "around and around and around" in a circle. You can take regular craft glue and "squeeeeeze" it onto the paper; you can "shake shake shake" (whispered) the glitter on, and take a paint brush and "dip dip dip" it

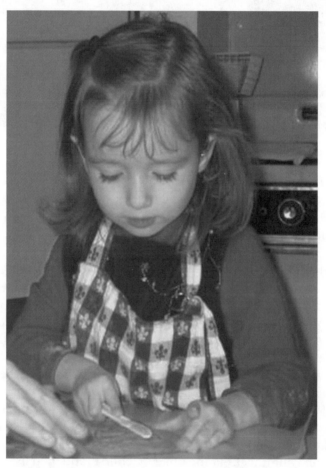

Figure 8–6. Megan is making cookies and listening to directions without watching the speaker; she's too busy.

in the water, or use stickers and "peeeeel" off the paper and "push" (whispered) the sticker on the paper.

All activities can be turned into listening activities. It just takes some creativity and thought as to how to target an appropriate skill and utilize your strategies.

Many children who receive CIs have the potential to develop spoken communication skills. Your child's ultimate benefit from the CI will be affected by the factors discussed at the beginning of this chapter. While no single approach is right for all children, many of the general principles of the Auditory-Verbal approach are essential for children who receive CIs if they are to reach their fullest listening potential. Listening is a learned skill and there is a hierarchy of development. Regular intervention with a knowledgeable professional, use of the listed strategies while keeping the listening hierarchy in mind, along with the incorporation of these strategies into your daily routines will help your child to reach his fullest listening potential. So, "live out loud!"

References

Colletti, V., Carner, M., Miorelli, V., Guida, M., Colletti, L., & Fiorino, F. G. (2005). Cochlear implantation at under 12 months: Report on 10 patients. *Laryngoscope, 115*, 445–449.

Dettman, S. J., Pinder, D., Briggs, R. J., Dowell, R. C., & Leigh, J. R. (2007). Communication development in children who receive the cochlear implant younger than 12 months: Risks versus benefits. *Ear and Hearing, 28*(Suppl. 2), 11s–18s.

Erber, N. (1982). *Auditory training.* Washington, DC: Alexander Graham Bell Association for the Deaf and Hard of Hearing.

Estabrooks, W. (2000). Auditory-Verbal practice. *The Listener, Summer* (Special Edition), 6–29.

Estabrooks, W. (2006). *Auditory-Verbal therapy and practice.* Washington, DC: Alexander Graham Bell Association for the Deaf.

Holt, R. F. & Kirk, K. I. (2005). Speech and language development in cognitively delayed children with cochlear implants. *Ear and Hearing, 26* (2): 132–148.

Kirk, K. I., Miyamoto, R., Lento, C., Ying, E., O'Neill, T., & Fears, B. (2002). Effects of age at implantation in young children. *Annals of Otology, Rhinology and Laryngology, 189*(Suppl.), 69–73.

Ling, D. (1989). *Foundations of spoken language for hearing impaired children*. Washington, DC: Alexander Graham Bell Association for the Deaf and Hard of Hearing.

Ling, D. (2002). *Speech and the hearing impaired child* (2nd ed.). Washington, DC: Alexander Graham Bell Association for the Deaf and Hard of Hearing.

Robbins, A., Koch, D., Osberger, M., Zimmerman-Phillips, S., & Rabin, L. (2004). Effect of age at cochlear implantation on auditory skill development in infants and toddlers. *Archives of Otolaryngology Head & Neck Surgery*, *130*, 570-574.

Schwartz, S. (2007). *Choices in deafness: A parents' guide to communication options* (3rd ed.). Bethesda, MD: Woodbine House.

Sharma, A., Martin, K., Roland, P., Bauer, P., Sweeney, M. H., & Gilley, P. (2005). P1 latency as a biomarker for central auditory development in children with hearing impairment. *Journal of the American Academy of Audiology*, *16*, 564-573.

Sindrey, D. (1997). *Listening games for littles* (2nd ed.). London, Canada: Word Play Publications.

Tobey, E., Rekart, D., Buckley, K., & Geers, A. (2004). Mode of communication and classroom placement impact on speech intelligibility. *Archives of Otolaryngology Head & Neck Surgery*, *130*, 639-643.

Megan's Story

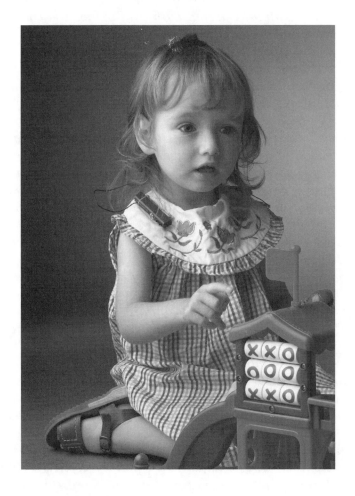

Megan passed an ABR at birth with normal hearing and soon began responding to our voices and environmental sounds. About 6 months later, I noticed that Megan quit responding to our voices, she quit requesting that we turn on her mobile, and she quit the babbling she'd recently begun. I knew she wasn't hearing even though friends and family insisted her hearing was fine. . . .

Megan's left ear was implanted 2 days after her 1st birthday. We immediately began working with a certified Auditory-Verbal therapist weekly, and we continued to work daily with Megan at home. Listening activities became an integral and relentless part *of our daily lives. Within 9 months of stimulation she understood simple questions and answered with "ya" or "no." She consistently used "Mama" and "Daddy" appropriately. She imitated words on command and could imitate pitch and duration as well. Megan used the Learning to Listen Sounds to label and request objects. She also began putting two words together (more bubbles). One year after implantation, at 2 years of age, Megan had an expressive vocabulary of 53 words and a receptive vocabulary of about 150. She followed a variety of one-step commands and demonstrated comprehension of several action words.*

Her right ear was implanted 1 day after her 2nd birthday. When only wearing her right implant she did not respond to her name or environmental sounds and her vocalizations were very limited. In an effort to catch up Megan's right ear to her left, we proceeded by using only her new implant for 2 hours per day. The rest of the day she used both.

Megan showed an immediate regression in her expressive vocabulary. She went from using 53 words to using 8. She did not show any regression in her receptive vocabulary; in fact, is seemed to continue to grow at a rapid rate. It is believed that the regression was due to an adjustment period, as she became used to listening with both ears. Within a month she was responding to sound and vocalizing almost as much with her right implant alone as when using both together. The time with only her right implant was reduced to 1 hour per day, and within 2 months we began having her use both implants together all of the time.

Megan's expressive vocabulary returned, and within 3 months of stimulation of the right implant, she had a receptive vocabulary list of 337 words, and an expressive list of 87 words/phrases.

At 3 years of age, 2 years after her first implant, Megan's expressive and receptive vocabulary has grown at such a rate that we are no longer able to track it. She uses six-word sentences consistently and is beginning to use some nine-word sentences. She comprehends and carries out commands with two critical elements. She asks, "Why," "Where," "What are you doing?" and "How come?" Megan consistently identifies toys, foods, clothing, objects, animals, and body parts and understands action words. She comprehends and uses location words, quantity concepts, and numbers. Her most recent testing shows her language skills to be within the normal range for her chronological age. Megan's bilaterally aided audio-

gram shows consistent response to speech sounds at the 20 dB level. She is enrolled in a mainstream preschool, and unless you saw the implants, you would never know there is any difference between Megan and her classmates.

Chapter 9

Advocacy for Optimal Educational Arrangements

By Linda Thibodeau, Lindsay Bondurant, and Jessica Sullivan

The educational process for your child is an ongoing journey that begins in the home and continues as your child matures and ventures into settings outside the home. As you get farther along on this educational journey, it will be harder for you to direct its outcome because you will have less control over the input, environment, and structure of interaction between your child and the system. Hence, you will need to be a strong advocate on behalf of your child in order to receive the accommodations necessary for learning.

The thoughts and feelings you might be experiencing at this time have been described through an allegorical "Trip to Holland":

I am often asked to describe the experience of raising a child with a disability—to try to help people who have not shared that unique experience to understand it, to imagine how it would feel. It is like this . . .

When you're going to have a baby, it's like planning a fabulous vacation trip—to Italy. You buy a bunch of guide books and make your wonderful plans. The Coliseum. The Michelangelo David. The gondolas in Venice. You may learn some handy phrases in Italian. It's all very exciting.

After months of eager anticipation, the day finally arrives. You pack your bags and off you go. Several hours later, the plane lands. The stewardess comes in and says, "Welcome to Holland."

"*Holland*?!?" you say. "What do you mean Holland?? I signed up for Italy! I'm supposed to be in Italy. All my life I've dreamed of going to Italy."

But there's been a change in the flight plan. They've landed in Holland and there you must stay.

The important thing is that they haven't taken you to a horrible, disgusting, filthy place, full of pestilence, famine and disease. It's just a different place.

So you must go out and buy new guide books. And you must learn a whole new language. And you will meet a whole new group of people you would never have met.

It's just a *different* place. It's slower-paced than Italy, less flashy than Italy. But after you've been there for a while and you catch your breath, you look around . . . and you begin to notice that Holland has windmills . . . and Holland has tulips. Holland even has Rembrandts.

But everyone you know is busy coming and going from Italy . . . and they're all bragging about what a wonderful time they had there. And for the rest of your life, you will say "Yes, that's where I was supposed to go. That's what I had planned."

And the pain of that will never, ever, ever, *ever* go away . . . because the loss of that dream is a very, very significant loss.

But . . . if you spend your life mourning the fact that you didn't get to Italy, you may never be free to enjoy the very special, the very lovely things . . . about Holland. (by Emily Perl Kingsley, 1987. All rights reserved. Reprinted by permission of the author.)

Following the diagnosis of hearing loss, several people will begin to interact with you along your journey. In addition to the cochlear implant (CI) team, you should be referred to the educational services provided in your area. You will work with the team member or school to develop an intervention program that should account for your child's unique needs. However, at some time, your child may be the first child with a hearing impairment to be served in that environment. Therefore, you will need to be knowledgeable about the accommodations that facilitate your child's learning, legislation that supports access to these accommodations, and how to be a strong advocate for your child. Throughout your child's life, your advocacy efforts for his instruction will vary along a continuum from minimal, where everything is in place for optimal learning, to maximum, where you not only need to inform others of the effects of hearing loss, but also educate them regarding the accommodations and technology that your child requires.

You need to be equipped with information to become a strong advocate for your child's needs in the educational setting. Following a discussion of classroom accommodations below, an advocacy model will be reviewed. Many of the decisions are related to legislation enacted to improve services for children with hearing loss and other disabilities. With this information, you can proceed to requesting and, if needed, demanding, the best accommodations for your child to reduce the negative effects of noise, distance, and reverberation in typical classrooms that can interfere with learning.

Accommodations

Children with hearing loss face many challenges in the educational environment, regardless of the class size or the expertise of the teacher. Terms that refer to placement of children with disabilities in general education classrooms along with their nondisabled peers are *inclusive* and *mainstream*.

Whether your child will be served in a small classroom with specially-trained teachers or in the regular mainstream of education, factors such as room noise, distance from the teacher, and echoes in the room can cause great difficulties in understanding the teacher. When a request is made for some action to be taken to help your child learn, you are requesting an accommodation. These may include special seating in the classroom, support services for speech therapy or classroom instruction, or specific technology the school may provide.

A child with a hearing impairment will communicate best when there is minimal background noise. Therefore, having a relatively small class size is important in order to minimize noise. Generally, classes less than 20 students are suitable unless specialized communication is needed, in which case smaller classes of 5 to 6 students are ideal. Regardless of the class size, it is important that your child be seated fairly close to the teacher. When possible, your child should be seated so that his better ear is towards the teacher. Being seated on the first row is not necessary because it may cause unnecessary strain, as your child would be looking directly up at the teacher for facial cues.

Support may also be requested for assistance with communication skills or classroom instruction. You may ask for speech therapy to help your child improve speech and understanding. In addition, an itinerant teacher, or one who comes into the class once or twice a week, may provide assistance with new vocabulary introduced in the lessons or other concepts.

Even with preferential seating, additional support services, and small class size, children with hearing loss may still miss important information if the teacher walks away while talking or there is some unexpected noise. The accommodation that should be considered for all students with hearing impairment in noisy school classrooms is the use of assistive technology to improve the signal-to-noise ratio (making the sounds that need to be heard clearer compared to the level of unwanted noise). There are many options for technology the school may provide as described in the next section.

Technology in the Schools

In educational settings, the child with hearing impairment will most likely benefit from additional technology to overcome the effects of noise, reverberation, and distance. Because each of these factors can degrade speech recognition and interfere with learning, efforts to minimize them must begin early. To facilitate the acquisition of the assistive technology, contact your school several months before your child enrolls. In addition to classroom accommodations, such as preferential seating, small class size, and speech-language therapy, FM technology can increase your child's ability to hear the teacher and enhance the learning environment.

Most CIs and hearing aids are compatible with FM systems, which allow for significant improvements of speech recognition in noise. The FM system is a short-range broadcasting system similar to an FM radio station. The FM system consists of two main parts: the transmitter worn by the teacher and a receiver that can be interfaced with the CI worn by your child. Because of noise, reverberation, and distance, the high frequency sounds such as /f, t, th, s/ shown on the audiogram in Figure 9–1 will likely be missed. This may lead to language confusions such as those shown in Table 9–1. Figure 9–2 shows the beneficial

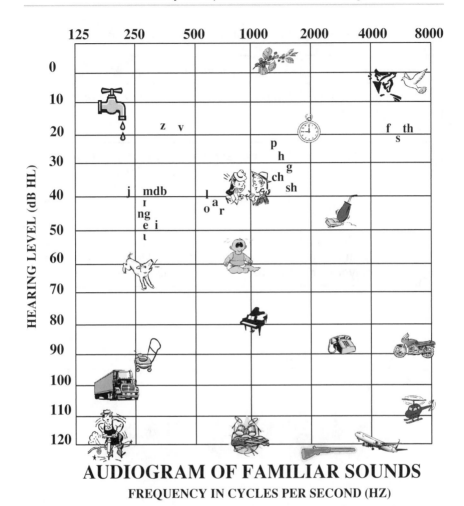

AUDIOGRAM OF FAMILIAR SOUNDS
FREQUENCY IN CYCLES PER SECOND (HZ)

Figure 9–1. Familiar sounds audiogram.

effects of using an FM system so that the signal is more perceptible in the noise. By placing a microphone on the teacher and delivering this signal directly to your child, the problems of noise and distance from the speaker are dramatically reduced. *Note:* It is important that the transmitter and receiver operate on the same channel; if they are not set properly or set without consideration of other FM systems in the school, your child may hear interference from other classrooms.

Table 9–1. Possible speech perception errors in a noisy classroom

	Context	Sentence Presented	Sentence Perceived
1	Cleaning up after free play time in centers	Time for snack!	Time for nap!
2	Near the fish tank	Can you feed the fish?	Can you read the wish?
3	Walking near the sink with cup of water	Take care, don't spill.	Take Cara the pill.
4	Talking with friend on the playground	Did you hurt your thumb?	Do you have some gum?

A. Listening with a cochlear implant in noise. Although some semblance of symbols can be seen in the noise, the meaning is not clear because the noise causes interference with receiving the signal.

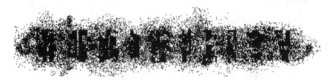

B. Listening with a cochlear implant in noise with an FM system. With the use of an FM system, the signal becomes more perceptible because it is more intense than the background signal.

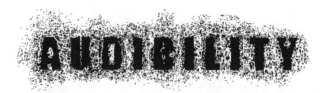

Figure 9–2. Visual analogy of speech perception in noise.

There are two main ways in which the FM signal may be received by a child with a CI. These include audio coupling, shown in Figure 9–3, and direct audio input (DAI), shown in Figure 9–4. With audio coupling, the teacher's voice is transmitted to a speaker that is placed near the student or mounted on the ceiling. With the DAI connection, the FM receiver attaches directly to the implant or hearing aid. This is preferable because the receiver moves with the child. Some argue that this is not the best connection because the teacher, or you, can't listen to the output (the electrical signal that is sent to the cochlea via

A. Personal Desktop System	B. Classroom Amplification System
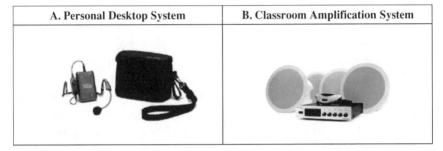	

Figure 9–3. Options for receiving the FM signal without direct connection to the CI. These systems can be either placed on the student's desk (A) or mounted on the walls or ceiling (B).

A. FM Transmitter	B. FM Receiver Connected to Cochlear Implants
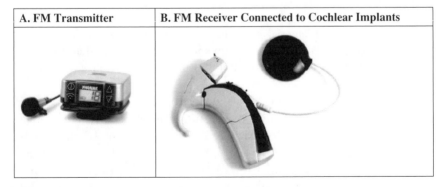	

Figure 9–4. FM systems consist of a transmitter worn by the teacher and a receiver worn by the student. In the left column is an FM transmitter by Phonak and Oticon, and in the right column is an FM receiver connected to the speech processor.

the implant's magnetic coil) to determine the quality of the signal. However, speech perception research with adults has shown that everyone benefited from using the FM system in a noisy classroom and performance returned to the level obtained with the CI used alone in quiet. If your child has limited language, careful informal assessment routines can be used to determine if the FM system is working and is not causing distortion. Withholding the optimal signal, on the basis that your child is unable to report the signal quality, is contradictory to putting on the implant itself. Young children who receive CIs often cannot verbalize the status of the implant signal. Therefore, the same routines used to establish that the CI is working can be used to verify that the child receives the FM signal.

It is very important that the settings in the CI be adjusted to operate with the FM system and that the settings are conveyed to the school audiologist, who is responsible for the equipment. Please remember that, in most cases, the school audiologist will not be able to change anything about your child's CI MAP, so ongoing communication between you, the implant audiologist, and the school audiologist is important. According to the American Speech-Language-Hearing Association (ASHA, 2006):

> With regard to cochlear implants, the regulations in IDEA (Individuals with Disabilities Education Act) now specifically state that MAPping is not a related service, and also clarifies that optimization does refer to MAPping a CI. Therefore, optimization services are not a covered service. Further, the language makes clear that a child with a CI or other surgically implanted medical device is entitled to those related services (e.g., speech and language services, audiology services) that are required for the child to benefit from special education, as determined by the child's individualized education program (IEP) team.

The implant audiologist needs to verify the connections to be sure that your child has the option of listening only to the teacher, or listening to the teacher while hearing classmates nearby. An audiologist should perform an evaluation to fit the FM to the CIs or hearing aid and ensure the settings on the FM receiver are optimal. Maximum benefit is received when there is a receiver on each side, whether it is two CIs, a CI and a hearing aid, or an implant and an FM system. The options that are available for the teacher's transmitter and for the student's receiver for the DAI option are listed in Table 9–2.

Table 9–2. Options for personal FM systems

Transmitter	Features
Microphone	The microphone may be small and clipped to one's shirt, fit over the head or ear to extend in front of the mouth, or built into the transmitter case and worn around the neck. Some transmitters have options for selecting the angle of reception from completely surround to a range of 45 degrees in front.
Charging	The power source may be rechargeable and have the option for using alkaline batteries if charging is not possible. Some may be charged through portable chargers that plug into car charging sockets.
Indicator Lights	There may be lights to indicate when the battery is running down or if there is no FM transmission.
Transmission Frequency	The channel or frequency of transmission may be fixed or variable. A *synthesized* transmitter can send a signal to change the channel on a synthesized receiver to match.
Audio Input Jacks	A transmitter may be connected to a sound source, such as a computer, to deliver sound to the FM receiver through the audio-input jack.
Receiver	Features
Style	Because of convenience, ear-level FM receivers are often preferred over body-worn FM receivers.
FM Ratio Settings	The FM receiver may be programmed or set with a screw driver to optimize the level of the signal from the FM transmitter relative to the level of the signal from the microphone of the CI or hearing aid.
Signal Options	FM receivers can be set to receive only the signal from the FM transmitter (FM setting), or that signal combined with the signal from the microphone on the hearing aid or implant (FM+M setting). CI users typically use FM+M setting to hear the teacher as well as the students nearby.

continues

Table 9–2. *continued*

Receiver	Features
Receiving Frequency	The channel or frequency of reception may be fixed or variable. A synthesized receiver, only available in ear-level receivers, allows for maximum flexibility in educational or community situations. The receiving frequency is typically fixed in body-worn receivers or may be changed in older body-worn receivers by placing the correct *receiving chip* or *oscillator* in place.
Charging	Some ear-level FM receivers draw current from the hearing aid or cochlear implant's batteries. However, they will drain more quickly when used to operate the FM system than when used just for the CI or the hearing aid.
Indicator Lights	Some FM receivers have indicator lights for battery drain and FM signal.

Once the FM equipment is selected and fitted, it is important to ensure that the teacher is instructed in the proper use of the microphone, care of the system, and charging of the components. Listening checks should be performed daily by using a listening earphone, if possible, as shown in Figure 9–5, or by connecting the receiver to a small speaker. Older children who are accurate reporters may simply perform the listening check with a peer who can talk into the teacher microphone while the CI student listens to the signal. It is important that the listening check include an evaluation of the CI microphone and of the FM microphone. After all components have been connected and turned on, the teacher checks the system by leaving the classroom and saying simple things like colors, numbers, or states. If the child correctly repeats the words, then the teacher places the FM microphone outside the classroom while it remains turned on and delivers speech to the child via the CI microphone. This check ensures the CI microphone remains active so that the child may hear classmates as well as the teacher. The signal from the teacher's transmitter

A. Listening Check via Earphone	B. Listening Check via External Speaker
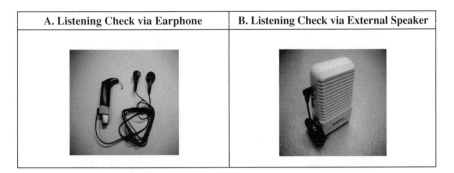	

Figure 9–5. The FM reception can be checked with most of the implants by Cochlear by using earphones (A) that connect into the processor or by using (B) an external speaker that connects only to the FM receiver.

will be significantly more intense so that it can be easily heard above the background noise. Involving other students in the daily checks is another way to facilitate social interaction for your child.

These accommodations can be critical components for your child's success. Therefore, knowledge of the process by which they can be obtained is important. A discussion of being an advocate for your child is presented next, followed by information regarding the steps one takes to request accommodations.

Advocacy Model

A generalized advocacy model is represented in Figure 9-6, where ultimately your child becomes the advocate! The foundation of this model is the information that must be shared with the many professionals who will interact with your child. This may involve sharing reports regarding your child's hearing loss, CIs, and hearing aids. However, if your child is functioning at a level to enter a mainstreamed environment where there are no special services for children with hearing loss, you may need to schedule a meeting to explain the effects of hearing loss and the technology your child needs to achieve optimal performance in the mainstreamed environment. This process may

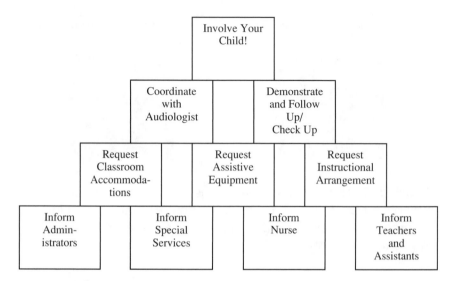

Figure 9–6. Advocacy model for parents of school-aged children with hearing loss.

involve showing the familiar sounds audiogram as shown in Figure 9-1 and playing various audio demonstrations from the Internet as suggested in Table 9-3.

When the information has been presented to the educational team, there will be a better understanding of the need for technology. When the need is understood, the acceptance and use of classroom accommodations and technology will increase. Your child's audiologist should be involved in the entire process so that communication can occur easily regarding the settings on the CIs and, if necessary, the hearing aid to interface with assistive technology. In addition to frequent communication, demonstration of the equipment is necessary so that all persons involved can use the equipment appropriately.

Finally, your child should be involved in as many steps as possible. For example, a 4-year-old CI user could be invited to show his teacher how the FM system attaches to the CI. A younger child may simply be asked to hand the teacher the FM transmitter. These actions may seem insignificant; however, they can deliver a strong message to your child that he is a part of the advocacy process now and will continue to be throughout life. Your child is interacting with peers who will also need to understand why the technology and accommodations are needed.

Table 9–3. Web resources to facilitate advocacy for your child

Audio Demonstrations	Web Resource
Audiogram and hearing loss	http://www.utdallas.edu/~thib/EARRINGFINAL/AudioDemos/Ed_Needs_Students_HL.ppt
Effects of hearing loss on speech	http://www.holmessafety.org/hlsim
Unfair spelling test	http://www.utdallas.edu/~thib/EARRINGFINAL/AudioDemos/Ed_Needs_Students_HL.ppt
Speech through a CI	http://www.utdallas.edu/~thib/EARRINGFINAL/EARRINGWEB_files/frame.htm
Benefits of FM systems	http://www.utdallas.edu/~thib/EARRINGFINAL/EARRINGWEB_files/frame.htm
Interfacing FM systems with CIs	http://www.phonak.com/professional/productsp/fm/fmconfigurator.htm
Information Regarding Services	**Web Resource**
Comprehensive information on disabilities	http://www.nichcy.org
State offices and programs	http://www.nichcy.org/StateAgencies/Pages/Default.aspx
IEP Conference Planning Kit	http://www.greatschools.net/cgi-bin/showarticle/2296
Individuals with Disabilities Education Act	http://www.fape.org/idea/index.htm http://www.idea.ed.gov/
General information regarding hearing loss	http://www.listen-up.org/index.html
John Tracy Clinic	http://www.jtc.org/
Resources and tools for early intervention	http://www.callier.utdallas.edu/txc.html

continues

Table 9–3. *continued*

Advocacy	Web Resource
Advocacy Incorporated	http://www.advocacyinc.org
A. G. Bell	http://www.agbell.org
Texas Connect	http://www.callier.utdallas.edu/txc.html
Wrightslaw	http://www.wrightslaw.com

Therefore, demonstrations can also be set up to explain why certain technology is needed and how it can benefit your child. This can be done in a way to increase your child's self-esteem. For example, your child's classmates might consider them the "lucky" one who might "overhear" special plans when the teacher forgets to turn off the transmitter while discussing a class party with an administrator in the office. Introducing the technology into the classroom can also be used to connect your child to peers by allowing him to choose someone to assist each week with battery, microphone, or charging checks. As you develop a strong "advocacy spirit," you will move through the educational decisions with confidence and positive outcomes for your child!

Educational Options

Preparing a child to enter into an educational system may be a significant and stressful time for all families, especially when the child has special needs. The communication and academic goals you have set for your child should be foremost in your mind when you are investigating the educational options. Discuss your goals with your audiologist, speech-language pathologist, and/or Auditory-Verbal therapist. They can provide information regarding the progress your child is making and assist you in making informed decisions along the educational journey.

Infants and Toddlers (Birth to 3 Years Old)

As you begin the early intervention process, it helps to familiarize yourself with some of your legal rights, protections, and responsibilities. The Individuals with Disabilities Education Act (IDEA) provides funding to states to assist in providing a Free and Appropriate Public Education (FAPE) to all children with disabilities, including hearing loss, in the least restrictive environment (LRE). The complete text of this legislation is on the Web site for the U.S. Department of Education (DEA, 2007b). IDEA provides legal guidelines for "birth to three" services through Part C, which was designed to address the needs not only of the infant/toddler with a disability, but also of the family.

In order to address your child's needs, a multidisciplinary team, including family members and professionals, will evaluate your child's performance and progress in a variety of areas, including physical, sensory, cognitive, and communication development (ASHA, 2007). If the results of the evaluation suggest that your child has developmental delays in any of these areas, a meeting will be held called the admission, review, and dismissal (ARD) meeting. Written notification of the meeting must be given in sufficient time for parents and all of the team members to be present. Parents are allowed to bring adult family members and advocates, and it is a good idea to have someone take notes during the meeting.

During the ARD meeting, a plan will be developed to address your child's needs through services that may include help dealing with CIs and assistive devices, physical, occupational, or speech therapy; nutrition support, and other services (including family support and case management). This plan is called the individual family service plan (IFSP) (Learning Disabilities Association of America, 2007). The plan must be reviewed at an annual ARD meeting to determine the appropriate goals for the next year of service.

For your infant or toddler, many of the early intervention services available will be home-based services. A provider, who may be a speech-language pathologist or deaf educator, will come to your home once or twice a week and teach you how to develop speech, language, and listening skills in your child's daily environment. These services may be offered through your local school district or through an Early Childhood Program. Because the instruction is demonstrated to the parent, the provider is often called a parent-infant advisor.

Preschool Children (3 to 5 Years Old)

If you are receiving services prior to your child's 3rd birthday, your parent-infant advisor should begin discussions of preschool options during the year preceding the transition. Before your transition meeting from a home-based to school-based program, you should visit all of the possible preschool options. At those visits, you should ask the teachers about their previous experience working with families of children with CIs and the types of accommodations that can be provided. Observe the classroom where your child may be placed and take note of the teacher-student ratio and the language level of the students in the classroom.

The type of educational placement you choose should coincide with the immediate and long-term goals you have determined for your child. The general classroom placements and descriptions are provided in Table 9–4. Language and communication needs must always be addressed when considering placement for children with hearing impairments. Before deciding on a particular placement for your child, the advantages and disadvantages must be explored. The only perfect placement is the one that fits with your child's needs and the goals for your family.

The transition from home-based to school-based programs may be confusing with the changing terminology and procedures. Once you've chosen a preschool program that best suits your child's needs, it is important to know your rights and options so that you can make informed decisions regarding your child's formal education. Children and youth (ages 3–21) receive special education and related services under IDEA Part B and the educational team will need to develop an individualized education plan (IEP) to replace the IFSP. Before the IEP can be developed, the local school district must determine eligibility for special education and related services. Additional testing in the areas related to the child's disability may also be requested. As defined in IDEA Section 300.301, the school system has 60 days from the time you give consent for testing to conduct the evaluation. The evaluation team will review all reports, including those from the assessment team, those you may provide, and current information from the parent-infant advisor to determine eligibility for a center-based program. In the event there is a disagreement with the results of the testing, you have the right to request an independent educational evaluation (IEE). The school district may be asked to pay for the IEE (Kupper, 2000).

Table 9–4. Classroom placements and descriptions

Placement	Description	Restrictive Level	Pro	Con
Self-Contained	Full time placement in a Deaf education with Deaf education teacher	High	Can be aural/oral or total communication	No normal language models
Inclusion	Regular education classroom with special education strategies and support services from Deaf education	Medium	Normal language models Team-teaching	Large student teacher ratio
Reverse Inclusion	Deaf education classroom with normal hearing peers as language models with a deaf education teacher	Medium	Normal language models Smaller student teacher ratio	May not be a general education curriculum
Mainstream	Regular classroom with general education teacher and possible services from itinerate deaf education teacher	Minimal	Normal language models General education curriculum	Must be able to work at grade level Fast pace

Once eligibility has been determined, you and the school personnel will develop the IEP for your child. This plan is reviewed and revised in the ARD meetings. The IEP team can consist of parents, a general education teacher, an audiologist, a speech-language pathologist, a deaf education teacher, and an administrator. Based on the recommendations of the professionals who have evaluated your child, a "draft" of IEP goals will be presented in the ARD meeting.

During the ARD meeting, goals can be added or removed from the IEP depending on what is appropriate for your child. Related services such as speech, audiology, and/or occupational therapy will also be discussed during this meeting. Once the IEP goals have been agreed upon, they will be effective for 1 year and the services can begin. It is a good idea to discuss with the teacher the mode of communication your child will use throughout the school year. Communicate with your child's teacher through weekly or daily e-mails or a journal where you can dialog in an informal manner regarding your child's progress throughout the school year.

School-Aged Children (5 to 21 Years Old)

As your child gets older, your focus will remain on finding an educational setting that best supports growth, learning, and achievement of academic skills. IDEA requires that the setting is the LRE, and, in many cases, the goal is that your child will attend the school he would attend if he did not have hearing loss (DEA, 2007a). IDEA does not require that every student with a disability be placed in an "inclusive" setting. School districts are required to provide a range of options to accommodate children's individual academic needs. These options are known as a "continuum of alternative placements" (DEA, 2007a). Any alternative placement you select for your child that is different from the regular education classroom setting should maximize opportunities for your child to interact with nondisabled peers to the extent appropriate to your child's abilities (ASHA, 2007).

Although a comprehensive evaluation will be conducted every 3 years, an ARD meeting will be held annually. During this meeting, your child's current performance and mastery of the current IEP will be reviewed. In addition, the accommodations and related services are also reviewed, as well as the presentation of the new IEP goals and services for the next year. Before the annual ARD, it is helpful to schedule a pre-ARD meeting with your child's teacher. At that time, you can informally discuss the progress of your child and review what will be discussed at the ARD meeting. If you have any concerns, you may also present them in writing and leave a copy with the teacher. This will provide you with documentation that you have expressed your concerns to the school personnel. It is important to remember that if, at any time, you think a change has occurred in your child's progress, you have the right to call a special review ARD meeting. For example, if your child was wearing hearing aids and then received a CI, you may want to call a special review because the goals or service may need to be altered accordingly.

As your child enters adolescence, you will want to encourage discussions about plans following high school. Options for college, vocational training, and/or employment may be explored with teachers, high school counselors, and private therapists who know your child. You will want to help your child determine postsecondary goals so that resources may be allocated to prepare your child to meet these goals. IDEA guidelines suggest that by the time your child turns 16, the IEP should include appropriate, measurable postsecondary goals based upon age-appropriate transition assessments related to training, education, and employment. In some cases, the IEP will include goals relative to independent living skills and the transition services (including courses of study) needed to assist your child.

Legislation

In addition to the provisions of IDEA discussed above, there are other legislative issues that are important as your child progresses through the educational system. It is helpful to be aware of these laws so you know how they may impact the educational services for your child or what options there may be, should you choose for your child not to be served in a public school by IDEA mandates. These laws include No Child Left Behind, Americans with Disabilities Act, and Section 504 of the Rehabilitation Act of 1973.

No Child Left Behind

Legislation passed in 2002, No Child Left Behind (NCLB), is intended to improve overall school performance by increasing standards of accountability. Given these results, parents are given some flexibility in choosing which schools their children will attend. To be eligible for federal funding, states must demonstrate the adequate progress of their students in certain grades through the assessment of basic skills. Because your child may need accommodations during these assessments, the team at your school that is responsible for the IEP will determine how the NCLB required assessments will be given. There are four options: (a) take the assessments with regular grade-level programs, (b) take the regular assessments with accommodations, such as extended time, (c) take alternate assessments based on grade-level achievement standards, or (d) take alternate assessments based on alternate achievement standards. The appropriate accommodations for the NCLB required assessments will be determined by the professionals who serve your child. If the accommodation alters the content of the assessment (such as in option d above), the scores cannot be included in the Annual Yearly Progress report for the school and the student would be reported as "not tested." It is critical that the usual services provided for your child are available during the testing. This includes the assistive technology described above. If the technology is not working or not available, the assessment must be rescheduled.

Americans with Disabilities Act of 1990 and Section 504 of the Rehabilitation Act of 1973

It is possible for a child to be ineligible for services offered under IDEA because of satisfactory performance at grade level. Some children with CIs are enrolled in regular classrooms in public schools and not labeled "auditorily impaired." In this situation, there are some applicable rights and protections under the Americans with Disabilities Act (ADA) of 1990 and Section 504 of the Rehabilitation Act of 1973. Both laws are aimed at prohibiting discrimination on the basis of disability. If a school receives federal funding, including IDEA funding, it is subject to these laws. Both laws define *disability* in terms of whether the person has an impairment that affects his ability to perform a major life activity; in this case, it applies to learning. Even if your child is not eligible for services under IDEA, Section 504 and ADA require that he be provided access to public places and programs. Schools may provide technology or schedule modifications to allow the student with hearing impairment access to the educational programs.

Application of Legislation to Children in Private Schools

If you choose a private school placement for your child, there are several issues to consider with regard to the public (IDEA funded) services available. If your child is already attending a private school and is not currently receiving IDEA services, either you or the school can request that the local school district conduct an eligibility evaluation as described in the previous section. If your child is found eligible and you choose to keep him enrolled in private school, the school district is not required to develop an IEP. However, the school district is required to work with a representative of the private school to formulate a *services plan*, which describes the specific services available to your child. As long as your child is a student enrolled in a nonpublic school, these services may be limited by the IDEA funding requirements.

On the other hand, if your child has already been found eligible for IDEA services and you choose to withdraw him from public school for placement in a private school, special requirements may apply. First, your child may be eligible for special education services similar to those described above. In some circumstances, it is possible to get the school district to reimburse you for private school tuition if the need for that placement can be demonstrated. There is also the potential of taking the assistive technology your child was using in the public school into the private school setting. It is also likely that the private school may provide the assistive technology under ADA or as it is required to meet private school accrediting regulations.

Many of these situations are complicated and may require the assistance of legal consultation. Resources for advocacy are included in Table 9–3. Much information may be obtained from the suggested Web sites, but if your questions cannot be answered through reading the information, a free service is available to parents of children with disabilities, known as Advocacy Incorporated. Its mission is to advocate for, protect, and advance the legal, human, and service rights of people with disabilities. It is important to remember that you are not alone in advocating for your child. Always include the professionals who are serving your child in your educational services concerns. They can attend the ARD meetings and provide support for the goals you have developed for your child.

Children with CIs have many opportunities to excel educationally. Because of legislation that provides a structure to access services in the schools, you can work together with educational personnel to develop the best plan for your child. The underlying strategy throughout this process is to start early so that information can be gathered for meetings, supportive personnel can be invited, and technology can be ordered and fitted appropriately. Until the process of children with CIs entering regular public school classrooms becomes more common, parents (you) will need to assist in educating others about their child's needs, as well as technology options.

References

American Speech-Language-Hearing Association. (2006). *ASHA cochlear implants IDEA issues brief.* Retrieved October 29, 2007, from http://www.asha.org/NR/rdonlyres/71772E44-FCCE-4FCB-8A8C-0788D698B03C/0/CochlearImplantsBrief.pdf

American Speech-Language-Hearing Association. (2007). *Status of state universal newborn and infant hearing screening legislation and laws.* Retrieved December 16, 2007, from http://www.asha.org/about/legislation-advocacy/state/issues/

Kingsley, E. P. (1987). A trip to Holland. Retrieved October 29, 2007, from http://www.our-kids.org/Archives/Holland.html.

Kupper, L. (2000). *A guide to individualized education program.* Washington DC: Office of Special Education and Rehabilitative Services, U.S. Department of Education.

Learning Disabilities Association of America. (2007). *Guidelines for the individualized family service plan (IFSP) under Part C of IDEA.* Retrieved October 29, 2007, from http://www.ldaamerica.org/aboutld/professionals/guidelines.asp

U.S. Department of Education, Office of Special Education and Rehabilitative Services (OSERS). (2007a). *Questions and answers on least restrictive environment (LRE) requirements of the IDEA.* Retrieved October 29, 2007, from http://www.wrightslaw.com/info/lre.index.htm

U.S. Department of Education. (2007b). *Building the legacy: IDEA 2004.* Retrieved October 29, 2007, from http://idea.ed.gov/

Chapter 10

Quality of Life Following Cochlear Implantation in Early Childhood

By Ann E. Geers and Christine H. Gustus

As the parent of a child with a significant hearing loss, you should know that her chances for a quality of life that resembles normal hearing age-mates are better today than ever before. Newborn hearing screening, early educational intervention, and use of hearing aids and cochlear implants (CIs) at young ages have all improved the deaf child's potential for successful social, academic, and vocational functioning within the hearing world. New developments in hearing technology and teaching approaches are intended to prepare your child to meet the challenges associated with early childhood deafness.

Challenges of Early Childhood Deafness

There are a number of challenges that may be associated with hearing loss and delayed language development. Children with hearing loss often develop vocabulary more slowly than hearing children their age, which may affect their ability to express their needs, thoughts, and feelings. They also may have difficulty understanding the feelings expressed by others. When they are young, difficulty expressing themselves may cause frustration, which can result in temper tantrums. From an early age, your child will be confronted with feelings that she cannot put into words. Difficulty expressing feelings, particularly anger and frustration, can result in greater impulsivity, "acting out," and other unpleasant behaviors. At somewhat older ages, children with hearing loss may not benefit much from opportunities for incidental learning, where information is learned by, for example, overhearing or just in passing conversation. When all communications must be directed specifically to a child, she can miss social and emotional content that hearing children receive with little effort from hearing the speech around them.

During the preschool and primary school years, children who can communicate effectively using speech are more successful in making friends and interacting socially with hearing age-mates. Some studies have reported that when children experience significant hearing loss, their language may be limited to literal expressions and concrete vocabulary. In such cases, a deaf child may have trouble with social interactions requiring complex mental strategies like foresight, anticipation, reflection, and imagination. For example, the child may find it difficult to see a situation from another person's point of view.

During the teenage years, young people are forming a sense of identity that will carry into their adult lives. Failure to develop a strong sense of identity is associated with low self-esteem and poor social adjustment. Some studies in the past have indicated that if a deaf child grows up in the Deaf community using sign language as the primary means of communication, she will develop a strong sense of identity with this community. Deaf children born into hearing families who do not sign have been reported to experience uncertainty about whether their identity lies with the Deaf or the hearing community. However, new research suggests that deaf children can develop a sense of identity in the hearing world and may identify with both hearing and Deaf communities. With new developments in early intervention and better hearing devices, positive self-esteem may go hand-in-hand with full participation in the hearing community.

Beneficial Effects of Early Intervention

Mastering a language and communication system as a child is a critical bridge to having a good quality of life in adulthood. Closing the language gap between deaf children and their hearing age-mates is one of the first steps in promoting not only academic competence but also healthy social and emotional development. While hearing aids and CIs do not restore normal hearing, there is evidence that they provide enough auditory stimulation to have a profound influence on spoken language development. The younger the child is when she receives a hearing instrument, the greater the benefit. Recent legislation mandates universal access to assessment of hearing in newborns. As a result, a significant number of children have had their deafness confirmed by 6 months of age. Early intervention programs can now provide hearing aids and, if appropriate, CIs at younger ages than ever before. Parent training can also be started when the child is at the very beginning stages of language development. Early intervention has a number of potential benefits for social and emotional development. Evidence indicates the younger the profoundly deaf child is when a CI is fitted, the smaller the language gap and the less "catching up" is required to achieve normal language levels. Early babbling and other vocal behavior that precedes spoken language development in hearing children have been found to develop normally in deaf infants who receive a CI as infants. This early auditory input stimulates the auditory parts of the brain and facilitates the development of listening and spoken language skills. In addition, it may influence children's ability to recognize the auditory signals of emotion carried by their mother's voice.

What are the long-term advantages of receiving a CI at a young age? Are deaf children and their parents satisfied with the CI after 5, 10, or even 15 years of use? What about the child's self-esteem and social skill development? Are CI users well integrated into the hearing world in terms of their academic, extracurricular, and vocational functioning? These are some of the questions we sought to address in nationwide studies of a representative sample of children with CIs. This research was funded by the U.S. National Institutes of Health.

Outcomes of Early Cochlear Implantation

A large-scale study of children who had received a CI during the preschool years (2, 3, or 4 years of age) was initiated in 1996. Most of the children had been deaf from birth, though some were born with normal hearing and became deaf within the first 2 years of life. The children had deafness as their only diagnosed disability. Both parents of these children spoke English as their primary language.

Children were invited to participate when they reached the early primary grades (8–9 years old). Over a 4-year period, 181 families from 33 different states and five Canadian provinces attended a summer research camp. All expenses were paid for the child with a CI and one parent to attend the camp in St. Louis, MO for 3 days of testing and recreation. During these 3 days, children were administered standardized tests in language, reading, and writing in the mornings and participated in a variety of planned recreation and fun activities in the afternoons and evenings (Figure 10-1). Our staff interacted with the children and their parents in social activities, engaged in conversations with them, and observed their interaction with each other. This gave us the opportunity not only to gather test scores and questionnaires, but also to gather more subjective information based on these interactions.

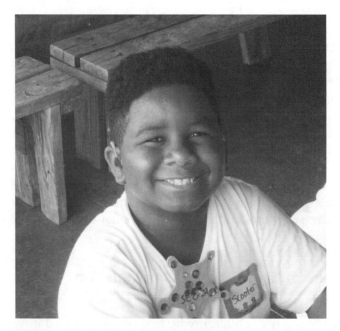

Figure 10–1. Scooter relaxes between activities at the Bill Gates Cowboy Ranch.

About half of the group of children came from educational programs that included sign language and half were in programs that used only spoken language. Some were enrolled in special education classrooms, while others were in mainstream classrooms; some were in public schools and others in private programs. This sample was judged to be representative of the wide range of educational and socioeconomic backgrounds that characterized children who received a CI between 1990 and 1996. These were some of the first children to receive a CI at such young ages. This large sample gave us the opportunity to see just how well the typical deaf child was adjusting, both personally and socially, after using a CI between 4 and 7 years.

In 2004, we began a follow-up study to retest these same children when they were in high school. This part of the study is still in progress, but so far 85 of the original group have returned to St. Louis as teenagers, which has allowed us to see how they are doing now that they have reached adolescence. In the following segments, we will describe the skills and achievements in language and reading as measured through standardized tests. We will also describe how they are getting along socially and emotionally as reported by their parents and themselves and as observed by our staff as they interacted with them in social activities during their time in St. Louis (Figure 10–2).

Academic Benefits

In the past, profoundly deaf students typically attended special education programs throughout elementary school and often into high school and college. Frequently this required residential placement, and deaf children lived apart from their families during the school year. Now, children who receive CIs at an early age are mainstreamed into classrooms with hearing age-mates in their neighborhood schools at younger ages than ever before. For many children, this means entering kindergarten at 5 or 6 years of age with age-appropriate language skills. Mainstream placement requires sufficient verbal, reading, and social skills to permit these children to integrate both academically and socially with hearing age-mates. Improved opportunities for independent action and responsibility that are associated with mainstream placement may have a positive influence on motivation and initiative in deaf children. The following summarizes the academic characteristics

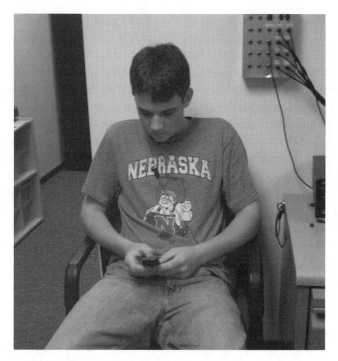

Figure 10–2. Trent is text messaging his friends while he waits to get his MAP tested.

of these children in the early primary grades and near the end of high school:

In early primary grades:

- 83% of the students were mainstreamed with hearing age-mates at least part of each day.
- 80% of parents reported their child was keeping up well with age-mates in school.
- 85% of parents reported satisfaction with their child's progress in school.
- 64% of the children scored within the average range for hearing students their age on a standardized verbal reasoning test.
- 52% achieved age-appropriate scores on a standardized reading test.

In high school:

- 95% of the students were mainstreamed for more than half of the school day.
- 85% were placed in the appropriate grade for their age.
- 74% reached age-appropriate levels on a standardized verbal reasoning test.
- 44% scored within the average range for their age in reading.

Auditory Benefits

Profoundly deaf students with CIs have been found to achieve substantially higher scores on auditory tests of word and sentence recognition than profoundly deaf students who use hearing aids. These tests measure students' ability to understand words and sentences through listening alone, using their CIs or hearing aids. In this study, students' listening scores continued to improve between 8 and 9 years of age and when they were 16 and 17. Their ability to recognize sentences improved from 59% to 77% correct. When we asked parents and children to describe CI benefits in everyday listening situations, here is what we learned.

In early primary grades:

- 95% of parents reported their child recognized her own name, familiar phrases, and the names of common objects without looking at the speaker.
- 55% reported that their child understood most of what other people said without looking.
- 36% reported their child could hold a conversation over the telephone.

In high school:

- 72% of students reported that they conversed on the telephone, at least with familiar people.
- 55% reported that they understood much of what is said on television without subtitles.
- 27% said they used listening to understand in their classes, without relying on lip-reading or signing interpreters.

One student who attended student council meetings wrote about her implant, "I love it. It truly helps me hear everything." Several teens discussed how they enjoyed listening to music with their CIs. One student reported; "I'm on the dance team at school. We do all kinds of dance —jazz, ballet, hip-hop—all of them."

Communication Benefits

Spoken communication reflects how well a child's speech is understood by others as well as the child's ability to understand others' speech. In general, children with hearing loss are more easily able to converse with familiar people than with casual acquaintances or strangers. Parents and students reported on their communication at both primary and high school ages:

In early primary grades:

- 75% of parents reported their child's speech was mostly or completely understood by familiar listeners such as the child's family, teachers, and close hearing friends.
- 60% of parents reported their child was understood by people the child saw once or twice a month such as relatives and neighbors.
- 50% of parents reported their child was understood by unfamiliar listeners such as waiters in restaurants and infrequent visitors.

In high school:

- 75% of students reported that they used speech exclusively when they went out in public.
- 78% said they understood the speech of the general public in stores and restaurants.
- 79% reported that their speech was usually understood by others.

Some students expressed pleasure with their ability to hear and speak as a result of the CI and others mentioned the importance of this benefit for their academic, social, or job performance. Students stated that they were pleased to have good oral communication skills so they could participate with their high school classmates in activities in their schools and communities.

Social Benefits

In the past, some studies of children with severe-to-profound hearing loss have identified difficulties in the areas of self-esteem, social-emotional adjustment, and family stress. In one study, as many as 50% of deaf children expressed concern about a lack of friendship and acceptance by others, as compared to only 16% of hearing children expressing such concerns. Other previous studies show that deaf children in mainstream classrooms have more trouble making friends and having positive interactions with hearing age-mates. Therefore, we asked parents and students about their social interactions in both primary and secondary grades.

In primary school:

- 70% of parents observed that their child's confidence improved following cochlear implantation.
- 85% of parents said their child is as independent as most other children the same age.
- 96% reported their child to be "a happy child and fun to be with."
- 82% reported that their child is talkative and sociable and makes friends easily.
- 88% said their child takes part in family relationships on an equal footing with other family members.
- 92% reported that their child played with normal hearing children at least once a week outside of the school day.
- 19% reported their child played with deaf children on a weekly basis outside of school.

In high school:

- 98% of the students reported having hearing friends.
- 79% reported having deaf friends.
- 98% of the students reported going to social events without their parents.

■ 88% scored within the average range for hearing age-mates on a standardized measure of social functioning, the Social Skills Rating Form. Ratings on the parent form yielded similar findings.

Self-Esteem

Self-esteem is a person's summary evaluation of her worthiness as a human being. This global human attribute has been shown to have a powerful impact on a person's learning, motivation, emotional well-being, and behavior. Good mental health is associated with positive self-esteem. Each child's self-esteem was evaluated when she was 8 or 9 years old with an adapted version of the Pictorial Scale of Perceived Competence and Social Acceptance for Young Children. The children were shown pictures and asked to rate feelings about their competence in a variety of areas, including physical, social, academic, and communicative skills. The majority of children exhibited a good self-image, with an average self-rating of 3.5 on a 4-point scale. As teenagers, the students completed the Rosenberg Self-Esteem Scale, in which they rated a set of 10 statements from strongly disagree (1) to strongly agree (4). Included were statements such as: "I feel that I am a person of worth, at least on an equal basis with others"; "I feel that I have a number of good qualities"; "I am able to do things as well as most other people." Sixty-five percent of the teenagers rated themselves at 3 or higher on most items. The remaining 35% had average ratings between 2 and 3. Thus, an overall positive self-esteem was maintained between primary and secondary grades by the majority of these CI users.

Overall Satisfaction with Cochlear Implantation

We asked the parents of 8- and 9-year-olds about their satisfaction with the results of cochlear implantation. In high school, we questioned the students themselves about their opinions regarding cochlear implantation. Here is what we learned.

In primary school:

■ 96% of parents chose an implant for their child so she would have a chance to be part of the hearing world (Figure 10–3).

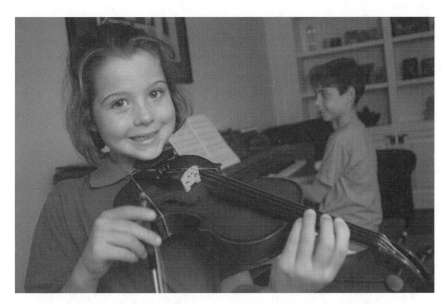

Figure 10–3. Emily's ability to hear music well enough to play music is not common among implant users. Some recipients, however, do hear well enough to play an instrument.

- 71% thought their child would learn to talk fluently.
- 86% thought it would improve job prospects in adulthood.
- 72% reported that their child's progress had already exceeded their expectations.

In high school:

- 80% of students reported wearing their implant virtually all waking hours.
- 20% reported wearing it some of the time.
- 90% of students indicated that they would have difficulty understanding the speech of others if they were not wearing their implant.
- 98% reported that if their implant broke they would want another one.
- 94% reported that they would strongly recommend a CI to the parent of a newly diagnosed deaf child.

One student wrote that parents should "get the surgery while the child is young . . . take the chance to help the child." Even those teens who frequently used sign language to communicate recommended the implant to parents of a young deaf child. As one student wrote, "I would recommend that a little deaf child has to get a cochlear implant so he/she could be successful." Another student commented that the ability to hear with her CI was "a wonderful, enriching experience of a lifetime."

Transition to Adulthood in Cochlear Implanted Teens

Extracurricular activities, sports, hobbies, and part-time jobs can provide adolescents with experiences they need to become self-reliant adults. In our study of teenagers, we were particularly interested in getting a picture of their participation in the life of their community, both in and out of the school setting. Most of the students (93%) were active participants in high school activities, sports, and clubs. The activities appeared to be as varied as those of any group of typical high school students. For the students who did not participate in an organized club, 92% were actively involved in sports or working at an outside job. Only 4% of the students did not identify an activity, sport, or job with which they were involved during the school day or after school hours. It is particularly interesting to examine the specific jobs, sports, hobbies, and clubs in which these teens participated.

Jobs

According to the information in the questionnaire completed by the teenagers, 51% held jobs while attending high school. This percentage is comparable to that reported for hearing teens by the Department of Labor Statistics. An estimated 49% of normal hearing teens between the ages of 16 and 19 years held jobs in 2006. The positions the teens with CIs held were wide ranging and appear to be the same types of jobs held by their normal hearing peers.

Seventeen percent of the students held positions that were provided by their family members, neighbors, or friends of the family. These jobs included such things as babysitting or cutting the grass at a relative's yard. As with most teens, these kinds of jobs would allow the student to earn spending money in a safe environment with familiar people.

Another category of jobs included those provided by individuals outside of the CI student's immediate circle of family and friends. The students' deafness did not appear to inhibit them from seeking and obtaining positions in many different areas. In most cases, the student was required to interview for the position, making spoken language skills quite beneficial. Some positions the students held required use of spoken language with the public. For example, several of the students worked in retail sales jobs that require communicating with customers in a store. Retail venues included a toy store, a parts store, a bagel shop, an art store, and a concession stand. One student used her oral communication skills working with children in a daycare setting, while another student taught figure skating to young children. One student proudly stated that she was a teacher aide at a summer school for "little kids," some of whom were deaf. Another student took advantage of her spoken language skills to work in a theater group. Other jobs included helping in a veterinary clinic, tutoring, and scorekeeping at sports events. One student stated that he was a lifeguard in the summer, a job requiring attention to the children and adults in the pool as well as the ability to communicate with patrons of the pool. Another student was a production assistant at a photographic company. He made the comment, "We communicate daily with almost no trouble."

Some of the other jobs listed did not require as much communication with the public. These jobs included bagging at a grocery store, working as a landscaper, cooking and serving food, and putting cabinets together. Several students expressed an interest in computers and one had found a position in data entry. Another student combined her interest in horses with a position working at the stable where she boarded her horse.

Activities and Clubs

Many of these students found time after school to join clubs and participate in a wide variety of activities. Some of the organizations required that the student be elected for membership based on outstanding academic performance. One student belonged to Mu Alpha Theta, a mathematics honor society. Several students were members of the National Honor Society (NHS). NHS inducts students into its membership each year who maintain a high gradepoint average and

exhibit leadership. Recently, the organization has added a require-
ment for community service hours in order to remain an active member. Some other teens in this survey were members of the Key Club,
another service organization for high school students noted for its
community service. Other students volunteered to work for Habitat
for Humanity.

Some clubs revolved around the students' political interests,
including the Young Republicans and the International Club. Participation in this type of club would likely require good listening and
public speaking skills. A number of clubs listed by these students,
such as Science Club and Space Camp, would require the teen to
speak at group meetings. One student was involved in the Junior Peer
Mentor organization, which required speaking to younger students.
Several of the students were members of the student government and
attended student council meetings. One student, who was a class del-
egate to the student council, also worked on the school newspaper.
She felt that she received great benefit from her implant and she
would recommend it to help students "function normally." Another
student was a member of the writing club and one was a member of
the yearbook staff. Participation in either of these clubs would require
excellent English language skills.

Some of the teens were in clubs that helped them pursue their
interests in the foreign language they were taking in school. Two students were in Spanish Club and two other students joined the French
Club in their high school, while another teen was in the Latin Club.
Other students joined clubs that helped them pursue special outside
interests. One student belonged to Future Farmers of America (FFA),
one joined a sorority in her high school, and another participated in
the Academic Band. Two students surveyed were members of the
drama club in their schools.

Many of the students belonged to clubs that focused on the sports
they enjoyed. These included soccer, rowing, curling, wrestling, track,
volleyball, figure skating, baseball, and basketball. Each of these activities would require the teen to take instruction and listen to rules or
directions from a coach. One student participated in tae kwan do and
martial arts. There were other clubs that that did not require much
spoken communication with others (magic club, knitting club, chess
club, fantasy card game club). One student mentioned that she belonged
to a deaf teen club in her city and another said she belonged to the
National Association for the Deaf. Several other teens were members

of sign language clubs associated with their high school. These students recommended the CI to families of deaf children. One stated, "Get the implant. Your child will most likely still interact with the Deaf world, but will be able to understand the hearing [world]."

Sports

Many of these students participated in organized sports in their high school or club sports in their communities. In the words of a typical teenage participant, "I play sports all the time. I play all the school sports—basketball, soccer, volleyball, and badminton."

The sports reported by students included the full range of team and individual sports available in most areas. Seventy-nine percent said they participated in a sport and the sports seemed to be a central part of their high school experience. The team sports that the students enjoyed included basketball, baseball (one boy reported receiving scholarship offers from colleges), football, volleyball, lacrosse, soccer, softball, cheerleading, and hockey (Figure 10–4). Each of these team sports would require taking instruction from a coach and some coaching from the sidelines. The ability to hear the coach's instructions with the CI would certainly be beneficial to the student in this setting.

The individual sports included track, horseback riding, cycling, swimming, tennis, golf, bowling, martial arts, weightlifting, figure skating, dirt bike racing, wrestling, motocross racing, and handball. With individual sports, the deaf teen would typically be participating alone and the coaching would occur mainly outside of the performance.

Hobbies

One of the favorite "hobbies" or activities of this group was hanging out or "chilling" with friends. Several students commented how much they liked talking on the phone and going to parties. As with most high school students, their friends play an important role in their lives. Many of these students with CIs mentioned they had hearing friends, so the ability to listen and talk with their CIs helped them become more integrated into the life of the "typical" high school student.

Other hobbies required group participation, like camping or boating with family and friends and shopping with friends at the mall. A few

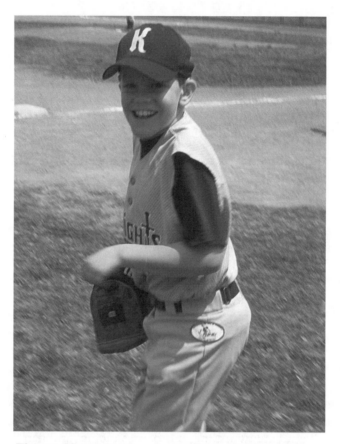

Figure 10–4. Andrew wears one CI and a hearing aid in the other ear. He enjoys all sports, but particularly baseball. He is seen here in his team uniform. Wearing the implant has not interfered with his playing.

students said they enjoy dancing and drama, activities that place considerable emphasis on listening and speaking. For several, participating in sports, such as soccer, sailing, rock climbing, four-wheeling, wrestling, and lacrosse, was listed as their hobby (Figure 10-5).

Several of the students expressed an interest in more solitary activities, such as reading and writing. Those who were more artistic listed drawing, making collages, making jewelry, photography, and scrapbooking, and still other hobbies listed were playing the guitar,

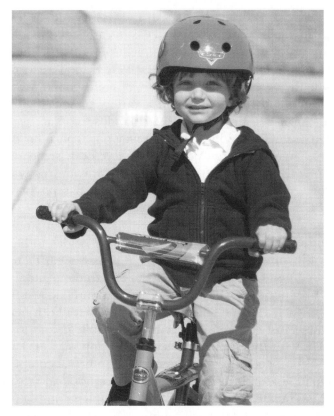

Figure 10–5. Ben rides his bike throughout the neighborhood with confidence because he wears a helmet, like all children should.

sewing, and "fixing things." One student said she enjoyed listening to music. She wrote, "I would say that an implant was a miracle to me. I couldn't live without it."

Like hearing teenagers, these students with CIs reported engaging in a number of hobbies that involve the use of a computer. The students said they enjoy playing video games such as X-Box and playing on the Internet. One student said he enjoyed "chatting on-line." Another student was active in "gaming" where several computers are playing each other in on-line games. In addition to these activities a number of students mentioned e-mailing and "texting" (text messaging on cell phones) with friends.

Life has changed dramatically in the past two decades for children who are deaf and who received CIs in early childhood. We had a unique opportunity to work with a large group of such children over a period of several days, first when they were 8 and 9 years of age and again when they were in their last years of high school. We were with these children and their parents in a variety of social situations, as well as in formal testing situations. This close contact gave us the opportunity to get to know them in a way not typical for those conducting research. The large quantity of data, both standardized and anecdotal, derived from these observations provides us with a truly realistic picture of how the students and their parents perceive the impact of CIs on the quality of their lives.

These data constitute a long-range view of what students with CIs can anticipate as they move from primary grades to high school and make the transition into adulthood. It is truly amazing to observe how typical these CI students appear. As one student summarized his high school experience, "I go to public school and I do just fine." Most of the teenagers reported feeling comfortable with both hearing and deaf friends. Most of them expect to go to college and to compete successfully with their hearing peers in the job market. Further follow-up will be needed to document their future accomplishments. We anticipate that improvements in early diagnosis and treatment of hearing loss, including younger cochlear implantation, advances in implant technology, and innovation in teaching techniques, will result in even further benefits for future generations of deaf children.

A Letter to the Doctor

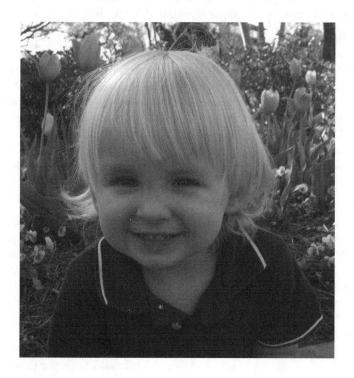

Below is a thank-you note to Brandon Isaacson, one of our cochlear implant team surgeons. As the letter explains, a year ago, Dr. Isaacson performed a complicated surgery on little Jordan, a hearing infant who survived meningitis but lost his hearing. Jordan's mom, Michelle, agreed to let us share this wonderful update with you:

Hello Dr. Isaacson! A year ago today, you spent a grueling eight hours in surgery with Jordan. He was a difficult and challenging case involving ossification, double array electrodes, etc. None of us really knew at the time whether or not the surgery would be successful, so we all just sort of held our breath and waited.

Fast forward to today . . . a year later. Jordan has around 700 words in his vocabulary (and probably more, but mom is really having a difficult time trying to keep up with all of the new additions). He is speaking in short phrases and sentences and is back on age level in his speech and language. He attends a mainstream preschool and doesn't seem to have trouble communicating with his teachers and peers. Some of my favorite words he now says are "noise," "sound," "listen," and, of course, "hear."

One of our biggest concerns when Jordan lost his hearing was whether or not he would ever be able to enjoy music again. Jordan is currently finishing up his second semester of Kindermusik class in which he sings, dances, and plays instruments. We have a small guitar for him at home which he plays on a daily basis (this is in addition to drums, harmonicas, maracas, bells, a horn . . . we are quite the music place around here!). Two of the CDs in my in dash CD changer are reserved for "Jordan music" . . . he is very insistent that I play "MMUUSSIIICCC" whenever we are in the car!! His favorite show continues to be "Jack's Big Music Show" and he is quite content to sit and watch the various music videos from the show which are broadcast on the Noggin website.

Jordan celebrated his third birthday a month ago. I became quite teary as everyone began to sing "Happy Birthday" . . . unlike last year, this year Jordan was able to hear the song . . . just awesome! In any event, I just wanted to take a few moments to reflect and to once again say thank you. If you ever have days in which you are feeling stressed/overwhelmed/wondering if what you do really matters, all you have to do is to think of Jordan to know that you have made a tremendous difference in Jordan's life and in our life as a family.

Many thanks again from the Capeners!
Todd, Michelle, and Jordan

Resources

Books

Apel, K., & Masterson, J. (2001). *Beyond baby talk.* Roseville, CA: Prima.

Chute, P., & Nevins, M. E. (2002). *The parents' guide to cochlear implants.* Washington, DC: Gallaudet University Press.

Chute, P., & Nevins, M. E. (2006). *School professionals working with children with cochlear implants.* San Diego, CA: Plural.

Cole, E. (1992). *Listening and talking: A guide to promoting spoken language in young hearing-impaired children.* Washington, DC: Alexander Graham Bell Association for the Deaf and Hard of Hearing.

Cole, E., & Flexer, C. (2007). *Children with hearing loss: Developing listening and talking.* San Diego, CA. Plural.

Estabrooks, W. (2002). *50 frequently asked questions about Auditory-Verbal therapy.* Toronto, Canada: Learning to Listen Foundation.

Estabrooks, W. (2003). *Songs for listening songs for life.* Washington, DC: Alexander Graham Bell Association for the Deaf and Hard of Hearing.

Estabrooks, W. (2006). *Auditory-Verbal therapy and practice.* Washington, DC: Alexander Graham Bell Association for the Deaf and Hard of Hearing.

Estabrooks, W., & Marlowe, J. (2000). *The baby is listening.* Washington, DC: Alexander Graham Bell Association for the Deaf and Hard of Hearing.

Koch, M. E. (1999). *Bringing sound to life: Principles and practices of cochlear implant rehabilitation.* Timonium, MD: York Press.

Ling, D. (1989). *Foundations of spoken language for hearing impaired children*. Washington, DC: Alexander Graham Bell Association for the Deaf and Heard of Hearing.

Ling, D. (2002). *Speech and the hearing impaired child* (2nd ed.). Washington, DC: Alexander Graham Bell Association for the Deaf and Hard of Hearing.

McClatchie, A., & Therres, M. (2003). *AuSpLan: Auditory speech and language.* Oakland, CA: Children's Hospital and Research Center at Oakland.

Moog, J. S., Biedenstein, J. J., & Davidson, L. S. (1995). *SPICE: Speech perception instructional curriculum and evaluation.* St. Louis, MO: Central Institute for the Deaf.

Pollack, D., Goldberg, D., & Caleffe-Schenck, N. (1997). *Educational audiology for the limited-hearing infant and preschooler: An Auditory-Verbal program*. Springfield, IL: Charles C. Thompson.

Robertson, L. (2000). *Literacy learning for children who are deaf or hard of hearing*. Washington, DC: Alexander Graham Bell Association for the Deaf and Hard of Hearing.

Rossi, K. (2003). *Learn to talk around the clock*. Washington, DC: Alexander Graham Bell Association for the Deaf and Hard of Hearing.

Schwartz, S. (2004). *The new language of toys* (3rd ed.). Bethesda, MD: Woodbine House.

Schwartz, S. (2007). *Choices in deafness: A parents' guide to communication options* (3rd ed.). Bethesda, MD: Woodbine House.

Sindrey, D. (1997). *Cochlear implant auditory training guidebook*. London, Canada: Word Play Publications.

Sindrey, D. (1997). *Listening games for littles* (2nd ed.). London, Canada: Word Play Publications.

Trelease, J. (2001). *The read aloud handbook*. New York: Penguin Books.

Wilkes, E. (1999). *Cottage acquisition scales for listening, language & speech*. San Antonio, TX: Sunshine Cottage School for Deaf Children.

Web Site Resource List

Alexander Graham Bell Association for the Deaf and Hard of Hearing
(A. G. Bell)
3417 Volta Place, NW, Washington, DC 20007
Voice: (800) HEAR-KID or (202) 337-5220, TTY: (202) 337-5221,
Fax: (202) 337-8314
E-mail: info@agbell.org
Web site: http://www.agbell.org

American Academy of Otolaryngology-Head and Neck Surgery
(AAO-HNS)
One Prince Street, Alexandria, VA 22314
Voice: (703) 836-4444, TTY: (703) 519-1585, Fax: (703) 683-5100
E-mail: webmaster@entnet.org
Web site: http://www.entnet.org

American Hearing Research Foundation
8 South Michigan Avenue, Suite #814, Chicago, IL 60603-4539
Voice: (312) 726-9670, Fax: (312) 726-9695

E-mail: ahrf@american-hearing.org
Web site: http://www.american-hearing.org

Auditory-Verbal Learning Institute
7205 N. Habana Avenue, Tampa, FL 33614
Voice: (813) 932-1184, Fax: (813) 932-9583, TTY: (813) 935-7944
E-mail: info@avli.org
Web site: http://www.avli.org

The Bionic Ear Institute
384-388 Albert Street, East Melbourne VIC 3002, Australia
Voice: +61 3 9667 7500, Fax: +61 3 9667 7518
E-mail: enquiries@bionicear.org
Web site: http://www.bionicear.org

Center for Disease Control and Prevention Early Hearing Detection
& Intervention (EHDI) Program
Mail-Stop E-88, 1600 Clifton Road, Atlanta, GA 30333
Voice/TTY: (404) 498-3032, Fax: (404) 498-3060
E-mail: ehdi@cdc.gov
Web site: http://www.cdc.gov/ncbddd/ehdi

CHID Database Search
CHID is a database produced by health-related agencies of the
Federal Government. This database provides titles, abstracts,
and availability information for health information and health
education resources. CHID lists a wealth of health promotion
and education materials, many of which are not indexed
elsewhere. Search the database using the term "cochlear
implants" to view citations to journal articles, audiovisual
materials, and books on this topic.
Web site: http://www.chid.nih.gov

Dallas Cochlear Implant Program
Web site: http://www.dcip.org

Deafness Research Foundation
641 Lexington Avenue, New York, NY 10022
Voice: (866) 454-3924, TTY: (888) 435-6104, Fax: (212) 328-9484
E-mail: info@drf.org
Web site: http://www.drf.org

The Ear Foundation
  Marjorie Sherman House, 83 Sherwin Road, Lenton Nottingham
    NG7 2FB, UK
  Voice: +0115 942 1985, Fax : +0115 924 9054
  Web site: http://www.earfoundation.org.uk

Food and Drug Administration (FDA)
  5600 Fishers Lane, Rockville, MD 20857
  Voice: (888) 463-6332
  Web site: http://www.fda.gov/cdrh/cochlear/index.html

House Ear Institute (HEI)
  2100 West Third Street, 5th Floor, Los Angeles, CA 90057
  Voice: (213) 483-4431, TTY: (213) 484-2642, Fax: (213) 483-8789
  E-mail: info@hei.org
  Web site: http://www.hei.org

John Tracy Clinic
  806 West Adams Blvd., Los Angeles, CA 90007
  Voice: (213) 748-5481, TTY: (213) 747-2924, Fax: (213) 749-1651
  Web site: http://www.jtc.org

Let Them Hear Foundation
  149 Commonwealth Drive, Suite 1014, Menlo Park, CA, 94025
  Voice: (877) 432-7435, Fax: (650) 617-2252
  Web site: http://www.letthemhear.org

My Baby's Hearing
  Helpful information for parents, including an extensive glossary
    section and a helpful question and answer section written by
    parents.
  Web site: http://www.babyhearing.org

National Institute on Deafness and Other Communication Disorders,
    National Institute of Health
  31 Center Drive, MSC 2320, Bethesda, MD 20892-2320
  Voice: (800) 241-1044, TTY: (800) 241-1055
  E-mail: nidcdinfo@nidcd.nih.gov
  Web site: http://www.nidcd.nih.gov

PubMed Database Search
PubMed is a database developed by the National Library of
Medicine, in conjunction with publishers of biomedical
literature. Search PubMed to access citations to journal articles
and, in some cases, find links to full-text journals. Search the
database using the term "cochlear implants."
Web site: http://www.ncbi.nlm.nih.gov/sites

Raising Deaf Kids, Behavioral Health Center
3440 Market Street, 4th floor, Philadelphia, PA 19104
Voice: (215) 590-7440, TTY: (215) 590-6817, Fax: (215) 590-1335
E-mail: info@raisingdeafkids.org
Web site: http://www.raisingdeafkids.org

Texas CONNECT
Educational materials and information for families with deaf or
hard of hearing young children. The site is produced by UT
Dallas/Callier.
Web site: http://www.callier.utdallas.edu/txc.html

UTD Callier Center for Communication Disorders
1966 Inwood Road, Dallas, TX 75235
Voice: (214) 905-3000, TTY: (214) 905-3005, Fax: (214) 905-3022
Web site: http://www.callier.utdallas.edu

The University of Texas Southwestern Medical Center Department
of Otolaryngology/Head and Neck Surgery
5323 Harry Hines Blvd., Dallas, TX 75390-9035
Patient phone: (214) 645-8898, academic phone: (214) 648-3102
Web site: http://www.utsouthwestern.edu/patientcare/
medicalservices/ent.html

Device Manufacturer List

Advanced Bionics
Mann Biomedical Park, 25129 Rye Canyon Loop, Valencia, CA 91355
Voice: (800) 678-2575, TTY: (800) 678-3575, Fax: (661) 362-1518
Web site: http://www.advancedbionics.com

Cochlear Americas
    400 Inverness Pkwy., Suite 400, Englewood, CO 80112
    Voice: (800) 523-5798, Fax: (303) 792-9025
    Web site: http://www.cochlearamericas.com

MED-EL Corporation
    2511 Old Cornwallis Road, Suite 100, Durham, NC 27713
    Voice: (888) 633-3524
    Web site: http://www.medel.com

Index